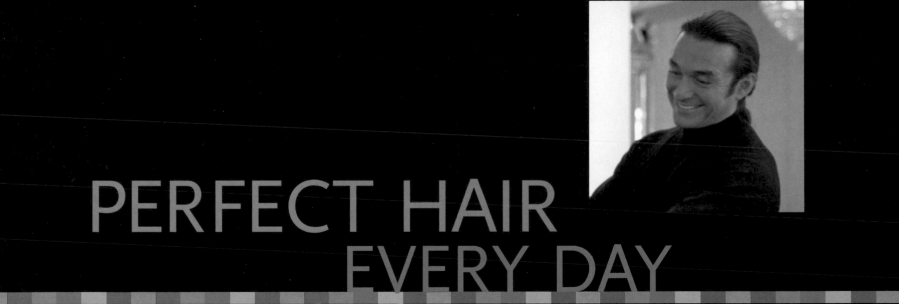

PERFECT HAIR
EVERY DAY

PUBLISHED BY QVC PUBLISHING, INC.
50 Main Street, Mt. Kisco, New York 10549

For QVC Publishing
Jill Cohen, Vice President and Publisher
Ellen Bruzelius, General Manager
Sarah Butterworth, Editorial Director
Cassandra Reynolds, Executive Assistant

A ROUNDTABLE PRESS BOOK

For Roundtable Press, Inc.
DIRECTORS: Julie Merberg, Marsha Melnick, Susan E. Meyer
PROJECT EDITOR: Meredith Wolf Schizer
BOOK DESIGN: Vertigo Design, NYC
COMPUTER PRODUCTION: Elissa Stein

Studio hairstyle and styling tools photography by Olivia Graham
Front cover and location photography by Jeremy Goldberg
Additonal photography by Gene Doton (page 8), Ehrlich Phtotography (page 14), K. C. Montgomery
(page 19), Kal Ye (page 5).

QVC Publishing books are available at special discounts when purchased in bulk for premiums and sales
promotions as well as for fund-raising or educational use. Special editions or book excerpts can be created to specification. For details, contact QVC Publishing, 50 Main Street, Suite 201, Mt. Kisco, NY 10549.

Manufactured in England
ISBN: 1-928998-36-4
First Edition
10 9 8 7 6 5 4 3 2 1

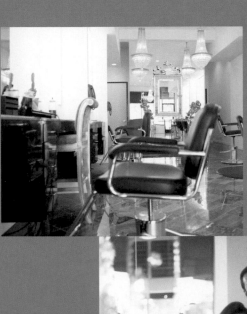

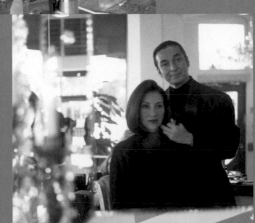

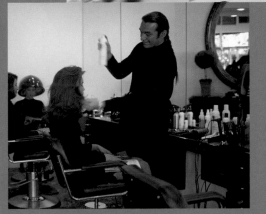

Acknowledgments

Mom, Dad, my family, and of course, the dear Lord, are first and foremost in my heart. A special thanks to my sister Sandra Chavez Hurley, who manages my salon beautifully, and to my staff, who make it a pleasure to work there.

My special thanks to my business partners Ken and Shelly Browning.

And thank you to Maria Shriver for her insightful inspiration.

I also wish to thank all the QVC producers and hosts, as well as the following people for their invaluable contributions to both my career and this book:

At QVC: Doug Briggs, Bob Ayd, Allen Burke, Donna Tarantino, Michelle Tacconelli, Michealann Vankirk.

Models: Carole Alston, Mandy Chavez, Trina Clark, Marisa Godoy, Sandra Chavez Hurley, Barbara Rexrode, Sioux Robbins, Robena Rogers, Louann Sheaffer, Ginny Trojan.

For QVC Publishing: Jill Cohen, Sarah Butterworth, Ellen Bruzelius, Cassandra Reynolds.

For Roundtable Press, Inc.: Julie Merberg, Meredith Wolf Schizer, Carol Spier, Carrie Glidden.

Business help: Morgan Hare, Natalie Di Lallo, Maria Camacho, Julie Groome, Sandra Chavez Hurley.

Hair and makeup assistants: Andres Velez, Marcia Bull, Jeanine Canter.

Last but certainly not least, I want to thank each and every one of my clients, all the QVC operators, and all our Perfect Plus customers who have made our enterprise such a huge success. I am what I am today because of you.

My promise to you

My promise is to show you how to style and take care of your hair the Nick Chavez way. I love pretty hair. I love hair that is clean and glossy, that smells great, and that feels wonderful to the touch. I love sensuous, rich-looking hair with plenty of volume—hair that moves when you move. And most of all, I love hairstyling that can be broken down into easy steps that anyone can duplicate.

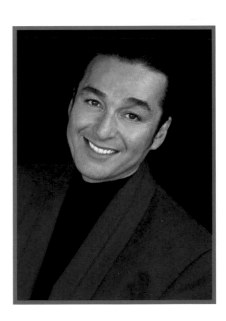

I know that if I can educate you on how to take care of your own hair as well (or nearly as well) as I can, I'm doing my job right. Many of my clients are amazed when they find out for the first time in their lives how well they can do their own hair.

I like helping women, and the best way I can do this is by showing them how to save time and money. Today's woman is very busy. She's taking care of her family, and she's working—so time is of the essence. Plus, it's very expensive to go to the hairdresser all the time. So whether I'm dealing with a client in my salon or with someone who calls in while I'm on television, I do the best I can to show her and tell her how to make the most of her beauty without spending too much precious time and money.

Most hairdressers don't want to give out their secrets, but as far as I'm concerned, take mine—they're yours. I've been truly blessed in my life, and I want to give back some of what has been given to me. I do this in my salon; I do it on television; and now I'm doing it here, for you, in this book. I know each of you will succeed!

Nick Chavez
Beverly Hills, California

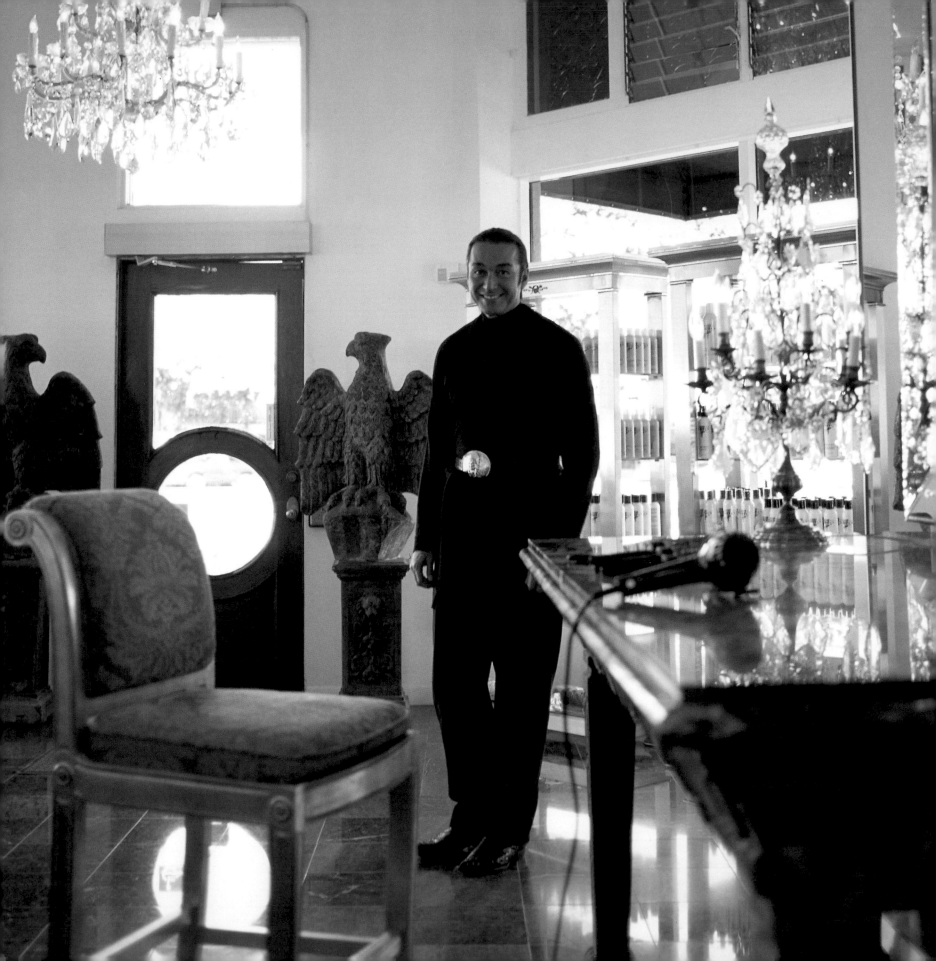

my life

I have had big dreams for as long as I can remember. Even as an eleven-year-old who groomed horses, cleaned out stables, and worked as a ranch hand after school because my family needed the money, I knew I was headed for something bigger and better. I didn't know exactly what, and I didn't know exactly how, but I did know that I was going to have to work hard to get there.

I come from a large Mexican American family (with Yaqui and Quechan Indian blood in there too), the second oldest of seven children—four girls and three boys. My siblings, from oldest to youngest, are John, Sue, Sonya, Joseph, Sandra, and Sherri. My parents, Kathryn and Juan, have been together for almost forty-five years, and as a family we are extraordinarily close and very proud of one another. The heroic Cesar Chavez, political activist and founder of the United Farm Workers union, was my third cousin.

My father is a farmer, and I grew up on a ranch outside Yuma, Arizona, in the Gila Valley. Like much of Arizona, it's desert terrain and the temperature can climb to 120°F during the summer. But I loved it then and I love it now, which is why I built a new home for my family there.

From horses to hairdressing

I started working with horses when I was about ten. I had a real love for them, and I used to eat, drink, and sleep horses. If you asked me then, I would have told you that I was going to be a horse trainer when I grew up. (Who knows? It could still happen.)

As a boy, I used to show horses (something I still do). I groomed my own, but we were too poor to afford the clippers I needed to clip the horses' whiskers, their ear hairs, and around the fetlocks. So I used to borrow some scissors from

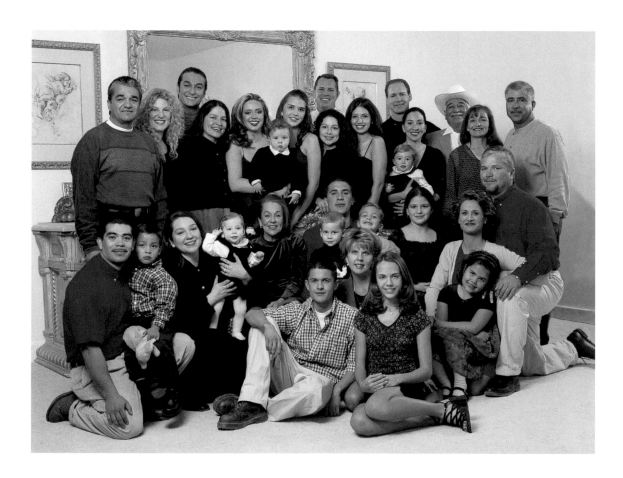

my mother's sewing box. After much practice, I got grooming down to a science and could actually trim the fine hair along the horses' ears without making any holes, which is extremely hard to do and takes hours with a very steady hand. I used to do it so well that no one would know I hadn't used the proper tools. I spent a lot of time teaching myself how to groom and braid so that the horses I worked on always had the most beautiful manes and tails.

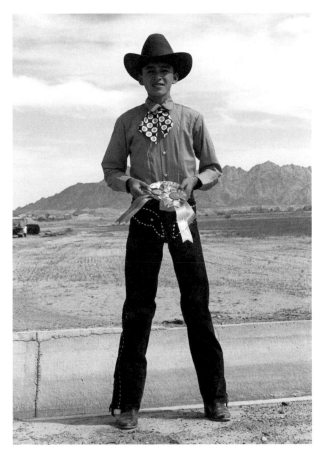

Grooming earned me the money I needed to keep and show my own horses and to pay the entry fees (and my brother John always helped me when I came up short). Before a show I'd get up very early, get my clients' horses ready, and then do my own.

In addition to showing horses, I also belonged to the 4H Club and the Future Farmers of America (FFA). These are clubs in agricultural communities in which kids raise their own prize livestock. Every spring we entered our animals in various competitions in which they were judged, and we sold them at auction at the county fair. I had my own lambs and cattle too. For the lambs I used to trim and card the wool so it would look nice and puffy. For my cattle I used to clean out the hair in their ears, trim their whiskers, and groom their coats to a great shine. (Elbow grease works wonders!)

What I learned on the horses, sheep, and cattle really started it all. I guess this means my hairdressing career actually began with those animals and my mother's little sewing scissors! The great thing about the animals was that they let me do my thing, and they never talked back. Boy, was I surprised when I came to Beverly Hills and started to do hair!

At around age fourteen, I thought to myself that if I could handle horses' manes and tails, I could certainly do people's hair too. My cousin Priscilla was my first "client," and I gave her a Farrah Fawcett-Majors cut. I had her running around with the hippest hairstyle in Yuma. Then I enlisted my cousin Gilbert and started doing layered haircuts on him.

Cousin by cousin, I figured out how to cut hair, and pretty soon I was doing my mom and brothers and sisters too. Then the word spread beyond the family. People in Yuma found out I could do hair; I would cut and blow-dry it for five dollars and give them something better than they'd ever had before. While still in high school, I built up quite a local clientele. I used to cut in our bathroom at home, and I remember my mom saying, "Nickie, you'd better clean up all the hair—your dad's coming home."

Initially, my father didn't really understand or support my passion for hairstyling. (He's come around since, I'm happy to say.) Coming from a Latin background, the last thing he wanted his son to be doing was styling hair. Because I was a farmer's boy, I was expected to make a career out of bailing hay, driving the combine, and digging ditches. But it didn't quite work out that way.

The move to Los Angeles

After graduating from high school, a friend of mine, Randi, and I decided to go to Los Angeles. We moved in with her mother, who was a banker in L.A. In exchange for room and board, I'd get up at five in the morning to do her mother's hair before work. Randi's mom introduced me to her friend who owned a salon on Sunset Boulevard in West Hollywood. The salon owner offered me a job at his place. It wasn't to do hair, though. Basically, I was a one-man cleaning crew and had to sweep up all the hair around the chairs, wash the floors, clean the bathrooms, and shampoo the clients. I was nineteen, new in town, and didn't have a hairdressing license, so my options were pretty limited.

One day the salon was extremely busy, and this girl came in off the street and said she needed to have her hair done. Every hairdresser in the place was booked. I went up to the owner and said, "I can do her hair." He looked at me and said, "Yeah, right." I begged him, "No, no, really I can. Give me a chance. Let me do her hair." Her name was Samantha, and she let me do her hair. I'll never forget my first professional hairdo: I teased her hair up and made a big, full bouffant. She loved it.

Samantha became a regular at the salon and would request me. She used to bring in her girlfriends too, and I'd give them all the big hairdos they liked. Samantha and her friends were my first clientele. The owner of the salon could not believe the work I was doing, because I had no formal training.

Before I knew it, I had built up my own list of steady customers. To make ends meet, I also worked at a clothing store (where I would hand out my card and tell people that I did hair too).

The other way I earned money was by winning dance competitions and working in a dance troupe that performed for fashion shows, charity events, and the like. I had always loved to dance and could hardly believe that I could actually get paid for it! This was right in the middle of the disco era, and my partner, Sarah Miles (not the British actress—*my* Sarah was American and had been a professional ballet dancer with a company in Paris), and I were an unbeatable combination. I had danced with a few different partners, but Sarah was by far the best technically and a joy to dance with. We competed everywhere and one year represented the state of California in the Playboy National Disco Championship, finishing in the top ten. I bought my first pickup truck with our winnings—a burgundy 1979 Chevy Silverado 4x4 with a short wheel base and a black interior—and boy was I proud of that truck!

From apprenticeship to the real deal

In 1977 I moved to a large salon in Beverly Hills, where I apprenticed until I became fully licensed. Then I was able to build up my own clientele. I used to get to work quite early and was one of the few employees who was there at 8:00 A.M. when the doors opened. I would always serve coffee, shampoo clients, and do whatever else I could. Eventually the women started saying (because most hair-dressers don't like to roll into work until ten), "Well, Nick can do my hair. He's here at eight o'clock." So I did blow-dries for a lot of those early-bird clients, who then started booking me for appointments for other times of the day as well. Word of mouth quickly filled my schedule.

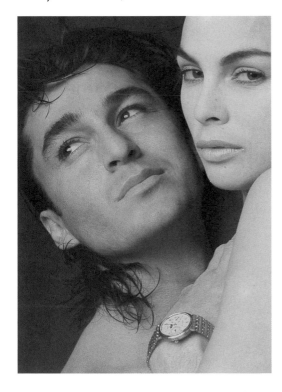

As a green kid from Yuma, though, I was still very shy. I wouldn't utter a word because I was so afraid I would say something stupid. You could never get me to talk. I would just listen to people, and I would do their hair. (Times have certainly changed; today you can't get me to shut up!) The difference between my small town in Arizona and the big city in southern California was like night and day. Where I came from, life was very simple and very easygoing; where I had landed in Beverly Hills, it was very busy, very fast-paced, and very intense.

At the same time, I felt right at home. I remember watching all the TV shows as a kid and saying, "I'm going to go to the Academy Awards, I'm going to go to the Emmys, I'm going to do all these things." My family used to look at me and think, "Oh my God, he's crazy!" I had all these visions of grandeur—I was sure that I was going to become somebody, even from an early age. When I was just a kid showing horses, people would tell my mom, "That kid's going to be a star."

Almost from the start (the late seventies and early eighties), I was working with stars. I did hair for a lot of young actresses from movies and television, as well as teen idols in the music business. Margeaux Hemingway, Dana Plato, Mindy Cohn and Kim Fields from the *Facts of Life,* and Lisa Hartman and Belinda Carlisle from the Go Go's, and Michael Damian from *The Young and the Restless* were all regular clients.

The life of an actor and model

In my late twenties I took a break from hairdressing. I had gone to Paris and, on a whim, walked into a modeling agency. By that afternoon the agency had me booked on some modeling jobs. Before I knew it, I was working as a model all over Europe—France, Italy, Germany, Switzerland—and ended up doing that for two years. I did runway for high-profile menswear collections (Yves St. Laurent,

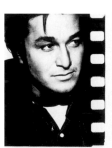
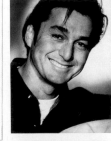
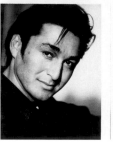
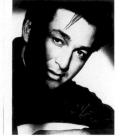

Thierry Mugler, Jean Paul Gaultier, Gianfranco Ferre, Valentino, and others); print work for all the major American and European glossy magazines including *Vogue, GQ, Elle,* and *Esquire;* and big ad campaigns for Swatch, Piaget, and many luxury goods manufacturers. At the same time I was the Jeff Hamilton model on a 100-foot billboard above Times Square in New York City.

Back in the States, I picked up a fair number of acting jobs, including a recurring role on *The Young and The Restless* and a featured role on a prime-time show called *Hollywood Detectives,* plus many commercials for such companies as Valvoline oil, Mazda Miata cars, and Taco Bell. By then my bashfulness was history—time has a way of healing shyness.

I hadn't exactly been regarded as actor or model material when I was growing up, though. As a child, I was so skinny I looked like a dead rat. They used to call me the human spring. When I'd walk down the halls in school, the other kids in school would call out, "Beep, beep!" because I had this big adam's apple and I looked like the Road Runner. But I always had a vision and I always had a sense of style. I was always different—totally, totally different—and I stood out like a sore thumb. After my modeling career took off, I realized that if big companies were spending millions of dollars on the clothes or the campaigns

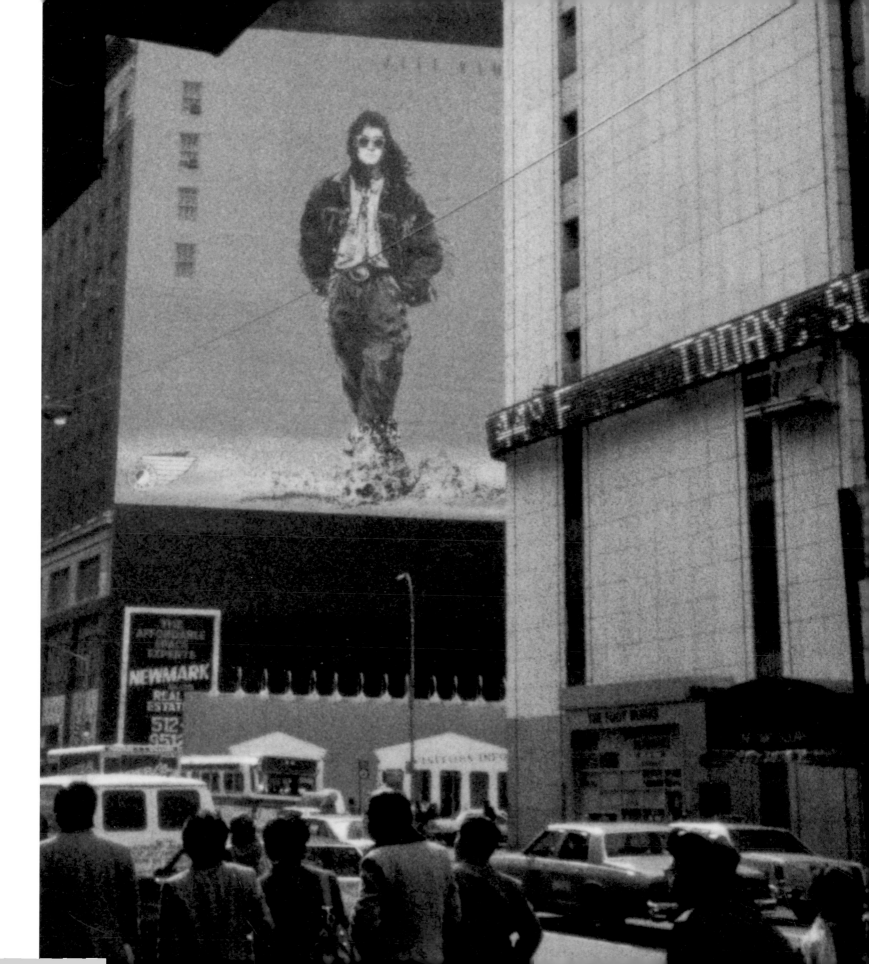

I was featured in, I must have something going for me in the looks department. Not bad for a Road Runner. *Beep, beep!*

As exciting as my life was at that time, I missed having a home base, and I missed working with hair. So it was back to Beverly Hills for me.

Perfect Plus is born

As my hairdressing skills gained versatility and my clientele increased, I began to notice the obvious: there were a lot of good hair-care products on the market, but no one (including me) was ever able to find a full line in which everything was great. Plus, there were about a thousand products out there, but they didn't necessarily work with one another. In fact, with the wrong combination of products, you could have a real disaster on your hands! I used to ask myself, why in the heck didn't somebody put it together and make the best of the best—the best hairspray, the best conditioner, the best shampoo, or whatever? So about seven years ago, that's exactly what I did. I gathered up all the best products I used every day, took them to chemists and manufacturers, put in more than my two cents, and said, "Make them better."

My mission was for my line to have it all. I wanted each product to enhance the others. I wanted something that would clean the scalp thoroughly but with-

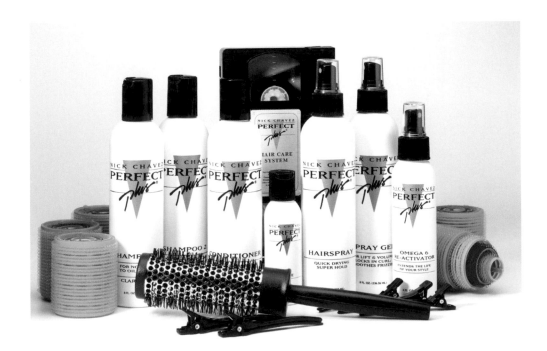

out stripping natural oils, because I knew that styling begins with a scalp that is super clean. Plus, I wanted a line that was going to work for every hair type and ethnicity. Everybody said, "That's impossible." And I kept saying, "No, it's not."

It took us over two years to get everything right for just the initial product launch. What I did as we were perfecting the line was to use the products every day on my clients. This turned out to be incredibly helpful. Since I'm blessed with such a huge clientele, I had every conceivable hair type in the world to gauge the results on. Having so many people try out the products made it very clear as to what was going to work and what wasn't.

The reason I called the line Perfect Plus was that I developed it as a perfect balance between ancient tradition and modern technology. I knew I wanted to include various herbal ingredients that had been handed down to me by both my grandmothers. My grandmother Virginia, for example, who is Quechan Indian, advised me to include aloe vera because it's such a wonderful healing agent and has been used by Native Americans in the Southwest for generations. At the same time, I hired the top cosmetic chemists in the industry to help us take advantage of technological breakthroughs.

Ultimately, it was really important to me that the line be affordable. My mom always used to say, "Remember to tell the truth, and make sure that everybody can afford it." Consequently, I priced Perfect Plus kits within everyone's reach and packed a lot of product into every deluxe kit, which includes Shampoo 1 Clarifier, Shampoo 2 Moisture Booster, Conditioner, Spray Gel, Hair Spray, Omega 6 ReActivator, Shine, 20 Self-Holding Rollers with 5 clips, my Salon Styling Brush, and an Instructional Video.

QVC enters the picture

As fate would have it, my business partner, Ken Browning, introduced me to an extraordinary woman who worked at QVC. Morgan Hare had until recently been a top executive at Avon and was well seasoned in the beauty business. She and I immediately hit it off, and she agreed to give me a ten-minute evening spot.

I went on QVC for the first time in August 1994. I had flown in a few days earlier to get to know the hosts and to do their hair before they went on. They loved the way their hair looked and talked about me on the air, which really got the viewing audience primed for my first appearance.

I had prayed to God and was confident we'd do well but was absolutely stunned at what happened because it all happened so fast. I went on air and boom! We sold out 1200 Deluxe Kits in just over two minutes. I could hardly believe it, and the look on my face must have been one of pure shock. Moments later, when it hit me, I ran to the phone to call my mom and dad and just started crying. What an amazing feeling that was, and I'll never forget it as long as I live.

Everything clicked, and from then on I was a QVC regular. And yes, when I can, I still style the hair for the female hosts, those wonderful women who gave me such a warm welcome in the beginning and still do.

On the set at QVC

I appear on QVC every six to eight weeks. The day before the broadcast, I travel from my home in Los Angeles to QVC headquarters in West Chester, Pennsylvania, where the shows are broadcast. I'm on for one or two days, depending on how we're scheduled, and we do two or three shows in a day. Some shows are an hour long; others are two-hour shows; and sometimes they give me fifteen-minute segments.

The pressure never lets up. Everything has to be absolutely perfect because we're on live. (It's not like you can make a mistake and take it back later!) For an 8:00 A.M. show, I have to be up by four-thirty or five. It takes me half an hour to get myself ready at the hotel and from there I go to the studio and immediately start working. I used to work alone but now I bring two assistants (Andres Velez and my niece Heather) with me from L.A. We get all the on-air models washed and blow-dried and get their hair set up and ready for whatever it is we're going to do. We're running nonstop right up until air time.

Between shows at QVC, we usually have production or new product meetings. If there's enough time, I go back to the hotel room to rest up or go antique shopping. (Stress relief doesn't get any better than a nineteenth-century painting, let me tell you!)

The schedule does get pretty crazy. I might do an hour show from one to two in the morning and then have to be up three hours later to prepare for a seven A.M. show the same day. In those cases I usually don't sleep. This means that I'm sometimes up and working for twenty hours or more. If it's a Today's Special Value (TSV), which runs for twenty-four hours, I'm up for forty hours or more. By the last show I'm so sleep deprived that I feel like there's mush in my mouth.

I try not to miss more than a day or two of work in my salon, so I catch the first flight back to L.A. after a broadcast or I take the earliest flight out the following morning. Sometimes I fly home, get off the plane, and go to the salon directly from the airport.

Behind the scenes the whole process is very intense, and it does get exhausting. This is where prayer comes in. When I pray to God to get me through, my energy gets going and the stress just falls away. Prayer is very much a part of my life on a daily basis. When somebody calls up on a show and mentions that she is fighting an illness or is in a difficult situation, I always say that I'll pray for her. And I do. That's for real.

The thing that's great about my shows is they have so much positive, life-affirming energy. They're a lot fun too and a pure adrenaline rush for me. I listen; I always talk with my audience, not at them; and I try to make everybody feel as good as they can about themselves. I just want to enhance what they already know and try to teach them how to work with their hair.

Opening up on my own

I had worked in a number of prominent salons in Beverly Hills, but I never wanted to open my own because I wasn't particularly interested in taking on the difficulties of running a service business. But about five years ago the opportunity presented itself in the form of a beautiful corner space with tons of natural light on a quiet residential boulevard in Beverly Hills. I couldn't resist, and within two weeks the Nick Chavez Salon was open. We opened so fast, in fact, that they were still laying the marble for the floors as we were doing hair (talk about an obstacle course!).

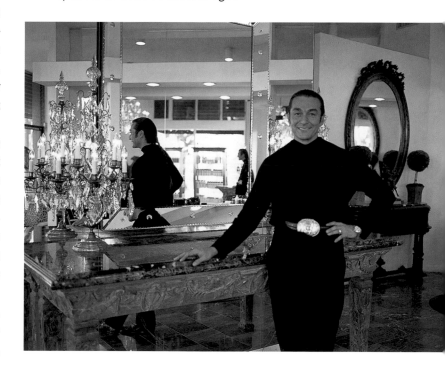

There are fourteen chairs in the salon, plus a separate color area. Eight hairdressers work there in addition to me, as well as two manicurists and two makeup artists. Last summer we completely renovated and decorated the space next door, and have created a beautiful makeup studio for my new makeup line.

My second-to-youngest sister, Sandra Chavez Hurley, runs the day-to-day operation of my salon business,

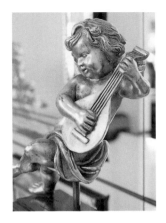

and she does it splendidly. My niece Heather Chavez is a shampoo assistant. And my brother-in-law Uriel Renteria works as Sandra's assistant. I'll tell you, nobody takes care of you like family.

My clientele is a very eclectic group of women and men. On the one hand, I've got the grandmother, mother, sister, and schoolteacher who are regulars. On the other hand, I've got a fair number of actresses and celebrities who come to me as well. And about 20 percent of the clientele is male. Once a woman becomes a regular client, it's just a matter of time before her husband starts booking his haircuts with us too. I'm dedicated to all my clients because they've encouraged and enabled me to become who I am. Listening to them, absorbing their advice and insight, has given me an education that money can't buy.

A typical day at the salon starts at eight in the morning, when we open. I live nearby and walk to work. I'm usually at work by seven forty-five and ready to go. We book appointments every half hour, and I have two assistants, Andres and Martha Hernandez, who help me keep things running smoothly.

On the average, I do twenty-five to thirty-five clients a day (up to forty-five during the holiday season). That sounds like a lot, but it's doable because I'm well organized. That, my ability to focus, and my faith in God have helped me build a career. I have a powerful sense of concentration and don't allow myself to get distracted from my goals, even if my goal at a particular moment is the blow-dry sitting in my chair who has an important lunch date in thirty minutes.

Everybody is amazed that I continue to work as hard as I do. They ask me why I still work in my salon when I could just do QVC and have a nice life. I always answer, "I look at going on QVC as going to the Olympics. And the reason I win the gold medal every time I go on QVC is because I train twelve to fourteen hours a day here in my salon."

Four days a week after work in the evenings, I work out with my trainer, Doug, at the gym. It's how I stay in shape and unwind after a long day. If I don't go out to dinner with family, I'm happy to eat tuna fish for dinner at home. (No kidding, I love the stuff and have had it for lunch every single day for the last twenty-four years.) On rare days off, if I can't be with my horses, nothing makes me happier than to wander around horse barns and antique stores. I love looking at beautiful things.

A day with the horses

The one thing that gets me away from everything is my horses. When I smell the animals and the grounds, I feel comfortable and connected to my past. Being with my horses takes me back to a time when all I lived for was horses, a very happy time of my life. All the tensions and stresses of the day are quickly erased by the profound sense of well-being these animals inspire in me.

I own about twenty-five quarterhorses and board them in San Diego. About once or twice a month on the weekend, I drive down there from L.A., ride all day, and come back. I am currently building my own training facility in Yuma, Arizona.

I participate in competitions run by the National Reining Horse Association. I don't get to show all that often, but my ranking has been in the top ten of my division, Amateur Reining. Essentially, reining is the Western version of dressage, and it is done in a riding ring. It involves a series of fast-paced precision moves and patterns on horseback, including figure eights, rollbacks, sliding stops, and high-

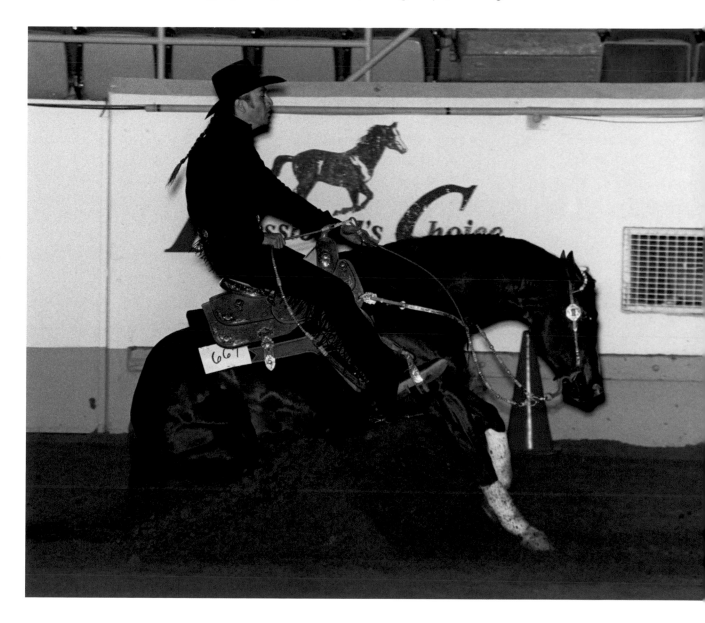

speed 360-degree turns in both directions. The whole routine lasts only about three minutes, but it's so intense that the three minutes last forever. Focus is the name of the game here, and until you've done it, you can't possibly imagine the amount of concentration reining requires.

Yvon Mathieu, who is French Canadian, trains my horses. Before competitions he hauls the horses all over the country in a trailer (which can end up being hundreds of miles away) and gets everything ready for me. I fly in the day of the competition, hop off the plane, get dressed (in full western attire, of course!), and show my horse.

I love all my horses. Just like people, they all have their own personalities. José, my sorrel stallion, is smart and sweet, whereas Lena, another stallion, is smart and intense. Then there's my mare Ashes, the mother of many of my other horses, who is—no other way to put it—a real little witch and very difficult. Having said that, though, Ashes is very bright and doesn't miss a trick (which just goes to show that no matter what your species, you don't want to mess with Mom).

As they have been since I was a boy, horses will always be an important part of my life. In fact, I'm planning to create a hair-care system for the manes and tails of horses that is really going to be something. Talk about getting back to my roots!

My approach to hairdressing

I am a very well-rounded hairdresser, and I color hair too. I started doing color work because I used to see the awful messes that would come into my chair—uneven, patchy application, blonde that was not gold enough, gold that was too brassy, white that looked gray—and I'd think, "I could fix that myself." So I perfected my technique for highlighting and hair coloring and for perming and relaxing hair too.

Not every hairdresser can cut and color, nor should they. But if you have a talent for both, the big advantage is that you can actually visualize the total look for a client, see how the cut and color complement each other, and work on finding the very best color to flatter the client's skin tone and the style to suit her taste.

I'm not scissors happy, so if you come to me, you don't have to worry that I'll cut your hair off. I won't give you some ridiculous hairdo that you can't duplicate yourself at home. I believe in giving you what *is* best for you, not what some magazine *says* is best for you.

Basically, what I do—and what I'm dedicated to doing—is to make women look pretty. I believe from the bottom of my heart that that's what women really want. When a woman feels pretty, she feels better about herself and the world around her.

Gratitude

Professionally, I know that I am very fortunate. I have a positive attitude, I always win, and I always set myself up to win. At the same time, I believe in telling the truth and being fair to make it a win/win situation for everybody I do business with. And I don't believe I have to make someone else wrong in order to make myself right.

The spirituality within me is my belief in God. I've learned that if something doesn't work out, don't worry too much because the Lord will always set you up with something that's going to work out even better. Personally, I know that I am blessed too. My family is wonderful, I have a very good life, I'm happy with what I've done, I'm excited about where I'm going, and I love what I do.

And for all of these things, there isn't a day that goes by when I don't express my gratitude to the Lord in my prayers.

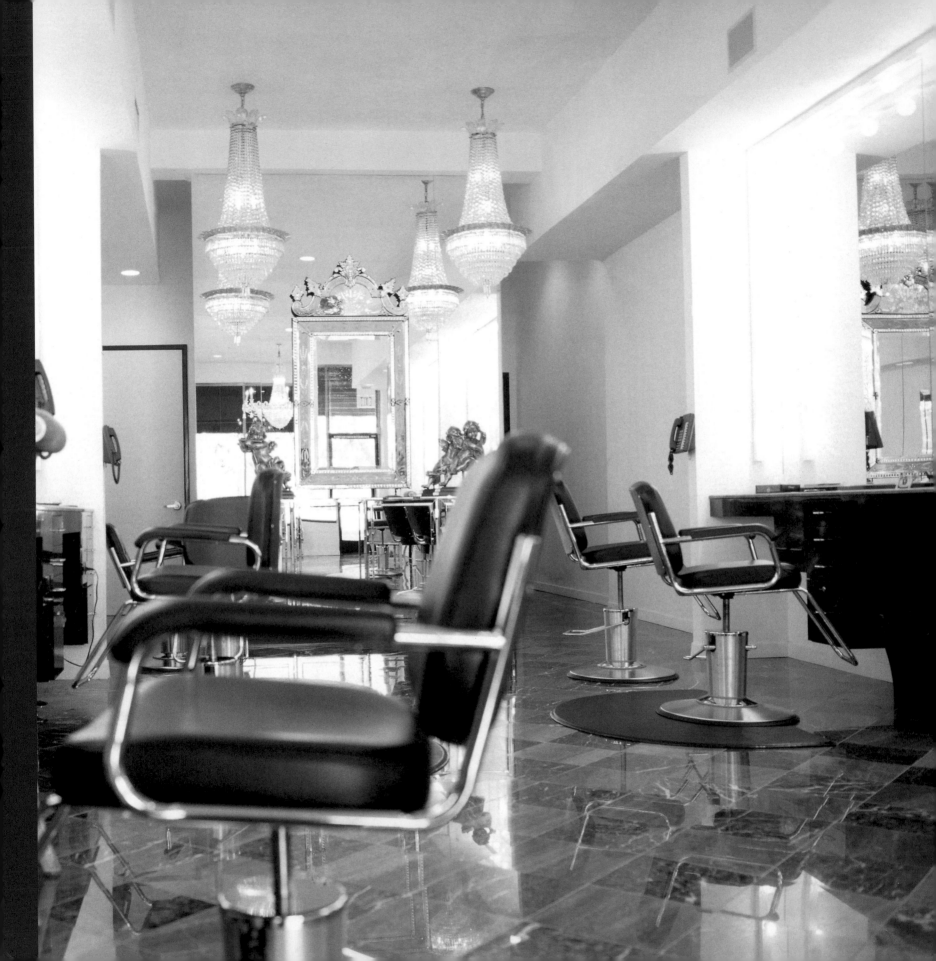

1

GETTING STARTED

you and
your hair

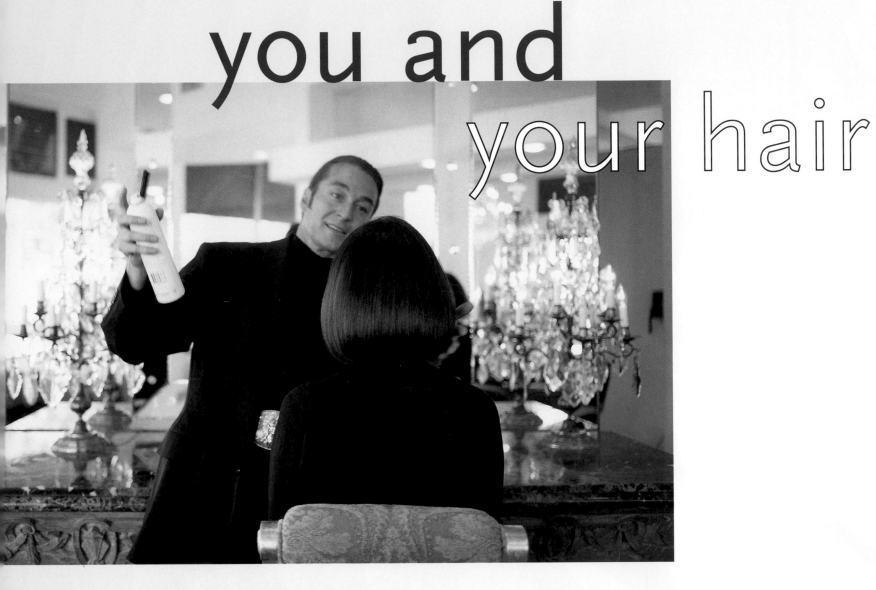

The same hairstyles don't necessarily work for all types of hair—what looks great with straight hair might not work at all for curly or kinky hair. But I'm going to make this easy for you. I've arranged the styling section in the last part of this book according to hair type so that you can learn precisely what styles work best with (or in the case of my salon, are the most requested for) your basic hair type.

When it comes to hair, why do we always want what we can't have? I have clients with heads full of curls who will do anything to get their hair stick straight and as flat as possible. At the same time, my clients with flat, straight hair constantly struggle to add fullness and body to theirs.

While you pretty much have to accept the hair you were given, the good news is that with proper product, blow-drying, and styling techniques, you can negotiate with nature a little bit. For example, I can't promise you thicker hair, but if you learn how to style your hair correctly, I can promise that it will look thicker and possibly even *feel* thicker. First, you have to determine your natural hair type and its texture and thickness, then factor in whatever else you've done to it.

Natural is what natural does

Of course, you probably have a pretty good idea already what your natural hair is all about. My definition of *natural* hair is what your hair is and what it does on its own when it air-dries after a shampoo without conditioner, styling products, or heat-styling. Natural also implies virgin hair that has not been colored, permed, or relaxed.

Whenever a new client sits in my chair, I run through my own mental checklist to categorize her hair. Of course, after twenty-four years in the business, I've got it down to a science, so that now it takes me only a minute. But I still do it, and it's this analysis, along with the client's input, of course, that helps me figure out what will work best for her.

Now let's work it out for you. Here's what you need to determine:

- Natural hair type—how much bend or curl is in the hair

- Natural hair texture—how smooth or frizzy the hair is

- Natural hair thickness—how much hair there is

- Present length—short, medium, long

- Present condition of the hair—shiny, dull, dry, damaged

- Types of damage, if any—mechanical styling, heat styling, chemical processing, environmental

- Your lifestyle—how nutrition, environment, and stress affect your hair

Many people have hair that tends to be a little frizzy or curly at the hairline, so don't make your assessment based on that. Your real hair type and texture begin about ¾ to 1 inch back from your forehead. Keep in mind too that hair analysis is often a matter of degrees. No one's hair is absolutely consistent all over her head (or for that matter, even along a single strand). This means that your hair may very well straddle a few categories. Be assured this isn't at all uncommon. Usually, though, one hair type and texture will predominate, and that's what we want to determine.

Think of the descriptions below not as absolutes, then, but as road maps to help guide you. For each category, note on an index card where you fit in and keep the card with this book for reference. Let's review the categories one by one to classify your hair.

Natural hair type

Hair type as we define it is how much wave or bend there is in your natural hair. When categorizing hair type, you'll notice that I frequently use the term *wave pattern*. Essentially, the wave pattern (or s-curl, as it is sometimes called) is how the waves or curls form as they grow out of the scalp. What we call a cowlick is actually a disruption of the normal wave pattern.

Straight hair

Hair strand dries straight and flat, with no bend. No wave pattern on the head. (Styling for straight hair begins on page 102.)

UPSIDE Shiny and smooth when healthy.

COMMON CONCERNS Flatness, limpness, lack of body, and possible difficulties curling it.

Wavy hair

Hair strand dries with a wave or a bend. Wave pattern usually lies flat on the head and can be loose or tight. (Styling for wavy hair begins on page 122.)

UPSIDE The most versatile hair type. Can easily be styled straight or curly, has lots of body.

COMMON CONCERNS A tendency to be uneven. The wave pattern is not necessarily consistent and may get frizzy or tighter at the nape of the neck.

Curly hair

Hair strand dries in a spiral or corkscrew, either tight or loose. Hair growth springs out and away from the head. Wave pattern is even and usually tight but can vary. Hair is 10 to 20 percent longer when wet, depending on curl tightness. (Styling for curly hair begins on page 134.)

UPSIDE Lots of body, fullness, and bounce. Blow-dries straight, with a lot of volume.

COMMON CONCERNS Inconsistency of curl size, uneven wave pattern, a tendency to frizz if handled too much, dry ends when chemically treated.

Kinky hair

Hair strand dries wiry. Erratic wave pattern grows out from the head and in different directions. No uniformity of curl. (Styling for kinky hair begins on page 148.)

UPSIDE Lots of body when blown dry correctly. Holds a style.

COMMON CONCERNS Gets frizzy and unmanageable, looks dry, ends break easily, requires heat-styling to control, might require chemical relaxing to soften the hair and make it more manageable.

Natural hair texture

Hair texture takes into account the degree of hair's smoothness, which has as much to do with how it feels as it does with how it looks.

Smooth

Smooth hair is shiny and feels silky and soft.

Frizzy

Nothing generates hair complaints the way frizz does. The term *frizzy* is a catch-all term for wild, wiry, fuzzy, rough-feeling hairs that go every which way. No matter what the cause of frizzy hair, the end result is the same for most . . . frustration.

Frizz can be the way the hair grows naturally, can be caused by chemical or mechanical damage, or may be the outcome of a serious underlying health problem. While the three types of frizz may look alike, they require slightly different handling, which can cause confusion when you are trying to figure out how to treat and style frizzy hair.

NATURAL FRIZZ Under a microscope, a frizzy strand of hair can look exactly like a curly one. The difference is that in a curl, the coiled hair loops together in a smooth unit. But with frizz, individual hairs fly out in all different directions. Frizz tends to be particularly common in curly and kinky hair, but no hair type is immune to it, particularly when the weather is humid or rainy. Then even some of the smoothest hair turns into bushy chaos. This is because frizzy hair absorbs or retains excess moisture, and in the process, it puffs up, expands, and just goes crazy.

HANDLING NATURAL FRIZZ Heat-styling, leave-in conditioners, and anti-humectant styling products (that is, those that repel moisture), such as shines, pomades, and serums, are best for taming frizz.

FRIZZ FROM DAMAGE This might look exactly like natural frizz: it's wiry, it pops out in every direction, and there's heck to pay when it's humid. While frizz as a result of damage (most commonly through aggressive chemical processes, such as hair coloring and bleaching, perms, and relaxing, or the overuse and abuse of heat-styling tools) behaves like natural frizz, the hair may also be fried, overly dry, and broken.

HANDLING FRIZZ FROM DAMAGE Hair that is damaged has a lot of porosity to it; that is, it absorbs moisture more easily because the protective structure of the shaft itself has been weakened. Frizz damage first requires a humectant to help moisturize and condition the hair at a structural level. Then, when the hair is styled, it needs gentle heat-styling to smooth it out, along with antihumectant styling products such as pomade to help calm the swelling of the hair and prevent it from absorbing environmental moisture.

Natural hair thickness

Hair thickness, also known as density, refers to how much hair grows out of your head. You might already know your hair thickness or else your hairdresser can tell you. Or, if you have long hair, an easy way to figure it out is with the ponytail test. Gather your hair into a ponytail at the nape of your neck. The diameter of the ponytail will tell you how thick your hair is.

notes on

THINNING HAIR

Every day I hear women in my salon declare, "Oh my gosh, my hair is falling out!" Thinning hair or hair loss is a huge problem, and I see a lot of it—in women as well as men. Hair growth is hormonally influenced, which is why hair is thickest during the teenage years and during pregnancy. At the same time, losing some hair is a natural by-product of growing older.

However, if you keep your scalp clean, style your hair correctly, use the right kind (and amounts) of products, protect your hair from the elements, and keep harmful chemical processes to a minimum, and you're still losing more than fifty to one hundred strands of hairs per day, you may have a problem that warrants medical attention. Hair loss can be a gradual process, or it may be triggered by a traumatic (either emotional or physiological) event. In some people, thinning hair is genetic; in others it comes from external sources. Sometimes hair loss is permanent; other times it is a temporary condition.

According to the American Academy of Dermatology (AAD), factors that can trigger accelerated hair loss or noticeable thinning include childbirth, high fever, severe infection or flu, thyroid abnormalities or disease, inadequate protein intake, medications, cancer treatment, birth control pills, inadequate iron intake, major surgery, fungus (ringworm) infection in the scalp, chronic illness, and stress. Furthermore, this kind of hair loss may not occur until several months after a specific event or condition.

A common type of hair loss called alopecia areata appears as totally smooth, round bald patches the size of a coin or larger. No one is exactly sure of the

Thin

Hair growth is sparse and you can see the scalp through it. The diameter of your ponytail is the size of a nickel or dime.

Medium

The diameter of your ponytail is the size of a quarter.

Thick

The diameter of your ponytail is the size of a silver dollar or larger.

cause of alopecia areata, but it is most common in those under thirty and in many cases the hair grows back spontaneously, without treatment. By far and away the most common source of thinning hair for people over forty is hereditary balding (androgenic alopecia or male pattern baldness). While most common in men, this type of genetic hair loss is not unusual in women. In men it shows up as a receding hairline in front and balding at the crown. In women, though, androgenic alopecia manifests itself as thinning over the front and top of the scalp, with the front hairline remaining fairly intact.

The most important thing to remember about thinning hair or hair loss is that if you think you are losing more hair than you should—for whatever reason—seek help from your doctor or a dermatologist immediately. The AAD emphasizes that the earlier hair loss is diagnosed, the more likely it is your treatment will succeed in encouraging regrowth. There are many medical treatments and techniques available to treat hair loss, and research in this area is ongoing.

Meanwhile, we've got to put some serious styling on your side. I'm not a doctor, and I don't prescribe. But I can show you how to keep your scalp clean and work with what you've got to give you the appearance of thicker, fuller hair. Volumizing products can help enormously in creating a richer illusion of thicker, fuller hair.

Since thin or thinning hair is such a concern for so many women, in Chapters 5–8, I've included specific notes on thin hair, targeted to each hair type.

Present length

Along with your hair type, the length of your locks determines what styles you'll be wearing.

Short

Anything cut above your ears.

Medium

From your chin to your shoulders.

Long

Past your shoulders.

Present condition of the hair

Once you've determined your natural hair type, texture, thickness, and length, it's time to evaluate the present condition of your hair. If it's not in tip-top shape, don't worry. I'll explain how to reverse, or at least manage, the problem.

The condition of your hair is determined both by what nature gave you and by what you have done to it in the meantime.

Shiny hair

Frizz-free hair that reflects light. If straight or wavy, the hair feels smooth and can flow through the fingers almost like liquid. In curly hair, the reflection bounces off the coils. Kinky hair can have shine too, but it's more difficult to achieve.

POSSIBLE CAUSES Youth, good genes, healthy living, proper hair care, the right styling products, careful heat-styling.

CARE AND HANDLING Keep doing whatever you're doing.

Dull hair

No reflective quality, shine, or gloss.

POSSIBLE CAUSES Improper washing and rinsing, product residue, harsh chemical processes, poor nutrition, underlying health issues, medication. While all unhealthy hair looks dull, it does not necessarily follow that all dull hair is unhealthy. It could just be the nature of your hair.

CARE AND HANDLING Proper washing with clarifying shampoos, rinsing, and blow-drying. Proper nutrition to build from within. Scalp massage, and exercise to increase circulation.

Dry hair

Dry, dull, and lifeless. Texture can be rough and strawlike or even so brittle that it breaks. It is not at all unusual to have dry hair with an oily scalp, particularly if there is damage involved.

POSSIBLE CAUSES Not enough oil from the scalp getting to the hair, naturally dry skin, damage from overprocessing and heat-styling, underlying health or hormonal issues.

CARE AND HANDLING Regular trims or cuts; moisturizing shampoos, conditioners, and protein-enriched treatment products; hair products with sunscreen; proper blow-drying technique; and air-drying when possible.

Damaged hair

Split ends, dry, discolored, brittle, lifeless, rough texture, porous, and may appear frizzy. Your natural hair type, texture, and thickness are what nature gave you. But whatever damage you see is a direct result of what you have done to your hair or in some cases is a reflection of how you live. First figure out what exactly the sources of the problems are. Then take action.

MECHANICAL-STYLING DAMAGE Hair loss caused by hair being tied when wet, pulled back too hard while styling, braided too severely, or exensions being improperly applied is called traction alopecia. It's not something to ignore, because if the pulling pressure is not relieved, it can cause permanent hair loss. This type of damage is characterized by breaking and thinning hair, particularly at the front hairline, sides, or along a part.

HANDLING MECHANICAL DAMAGE Gentler handling when drying and styling, looser styles, looser braids at the root, loosening extensions at the root, *never* sleeping with hair in an elastic band.

HEAT-STYLING DAMAGE Heat-styling—whether with a blow dryer, electric rollers, curling iron, flat iron, or crimping iron—runs neck and neck with chemical processing when it comes to damaging the hair. Just learning the proper technique for blow-drying hair could significantly reduce the amount of existing hair damage. Hair gets damaged when people hold the dryer too close; use too much of the wrong products; use heat-styling tools (other than the blow dryer) on wet hair, causing it to break off; and pull so hard with the round brush while blow-drying that the hair snaps off. Heat-damaged hair looks fried, dull, and brittle and has split ends and breakage.

HANDLING HEAT DAMAGE Regular trims and cuts, moisturizing hair-care products, regular conditioning treatments, blow-drying correctly without pulling unevenly, and air-drying when possible.

CHEMICAL-PROCESSING DAMAGE All chemically treated hair is damaged in some way because its structure has been forcibly altered. The idea behind a good chemical service, then, is to have it done (or do it yourself) skillfully and with as little damage as possible, so that the hair still seems healthy. (Sometimes a little damage can make the hair fuller and more manageable, but this depends on your hair type.) Hair that's chemically damaged looks fried, dull, and brittle and has split ends and breakage. Even if your hair looks wonderful, however, chemical processing means that the structure has been compromised, making the hair more porous, more fragile, much drier, and more prone to frizziness and breakage.

HANDLING CHEMICAL DAMAGE Regular trims and cuts, products for chemically treated hair, regular conditioning treatments, blow-drying correctly, air-drying when possible, making sure that when regrowth is touched up with color, it does not overlap with already treated hair, which would double the damage.

ENVIRONMENTAL DAMAGE The environment can do considerable harm to your hair if you don't take the proper precautions. Sun damage can cause bleached-out color; wind damage can cause breakage; weather extremes can cause dryness and dullness; salt water can cause bleached-out color, dryness, and porosity; chlorine can cause a green tinge to blonde hair, dried-out ends, brittleness, and porosity; and pollution can cause dullness.

HANDLING ENVIRONMENTAL DAMAGE Products with sunscreens; moisturizing products containing vitamins A, D, and C; clarifying shampoos (for salt and chlorine); application of protective conditioners and pomades before exposure to the sun, chlorine, and salt water.

Your lifestyle

Hair doesn't lie. Like it or not, your hair is a reflection of your quality of life and how well you take care of yourself. If you abuse your health—with junk food, with alcohol, with drugs—it will show in your hair. I'm not kidding when I say that living a healthy life is the first step to having beautiful, healthy hair. At the same time, don't deprive yourself too much. Too little fat in the diet can result in dry, dull hair. And be sure to relax! Stress—over time—may lead to accelerated hair loss.

Hair grows only about $1/2$ inch per month on average, so even if you change your life dramatically overnight, eat nothing but the right foods, drink plenty of water, exercise away your stress, and are in perfect health, it will still take months for these improvements to be reflected in your hair's condition. This may seem frustrating, but I say, "What are you waiting for? The sooner you get started, the sooner it will pay off." What you see now in your hair that you dislike (or do like, for that matter) is the result of years of behavior. It all adds up.

Hair color, relaxing, and perms

Hair color, relaxing, and perms are referred to as chemical services and the hairdresser who does one usually (although not always) has some experience with all three.

Chemical services are best left to professionals because the potential for mistakes is so great. And with volatile chemicals you run the risk not only of damaging your hair but of burning your scalp and scarring your skin. Consequently, in all good conscience I must ask you to use a professional hairdresser if you want relaxers or permanent waves.

As for hair color, anything beyond simple one-process (single-step) coloring is best left to the pros too. That includes double-process coloring (bleaching hair, then applying another color—usually blonde—on top), streaking, and highlights.

Hair color precautions

Here are a few things to keep in mind when coloring your hair:

- Sunscreens in shampoo, conditioners, and styling products help preserve the richness of hair color, while some dandruff shampoos will fade hair color.

- Never color your hair when your scalp is squeaky clean, or you risk burning your scalp. The best time to color hair is a day or two after shampooing. If you do have excess product buildup on your ends the day you are going to have it colored, wash the ends thoroughly without scrubbing the scalp.

- Make sure all hairspray and gel are washed out of your hair really well before coloring your hair. If you try to color hair with some styling product in it, you can end up with unattractive, uneven blotches.

- Even if it looks wonderful, remember that color-treated hair is damaged hair and, as such, should be handled with care and conditioned regularly. Use milder products or those specifically developed for color-treated hair.

Do-it-yourself one-process

If you do decide to color at home, be sure to use the gloves that are supplied. Also, apply a thin film of petroleum jelly around your hairline (but don't get it into the hair itself) so that the color doesn't end up staining your skin.

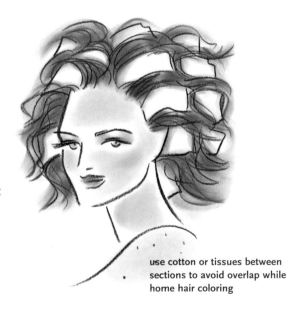

use cotton or tissues between sections to avoid overlap while home hair coloring

The most critical thing to avoid when coloring your hair at home (or in a salon) is overlapping. What I mean by overlapping is being sloppy and having one section of the hair lying on top of another. This will cause an uneven buildup of color. And if the hairdresser overlaps while streaking or bleaching your hair, it can also cause a lot of breakage.

Color your hair by working in even sections. Start by touching up the roots, and as you color them in each section, run a length of cotton or a rolled-up tissue between the sections so that the hair doesn't overlap on itself. Color should be left on the ends for five minutes maximum.

Handy hint: For more even coverage, moisten the ends of your hair before running color through it.

Gray news

When and how much you turn gray is genetically determined. Some people begin turning gray in their twenties, while others still have dark hair into their sixties. Generally, though, gray hair starts appearing in the thirties. The word *gray* actually isn't an accurate description because the pigment of the hair isn't gray or silver at all—it's white. And no, you can't turn gray overnight from stress or a bad fright.

Coloring, tinting, and dyeing (different words for the same thing) the hair are ways to restore color and luminosity to gray hair. Keeping your scalp clean and using the proper conditioning products also will enhance your hair to give it a more youthful quality.

Gray hair is more coarse, wiry, and resistant to color than other hair. Consequently, permanent hair color (versus semipermanent hair color) is the best choice to cover gray because of its holding power.

Choosing the right hair color to cover gray hair is an art in itself, and a professional with a good eye can help guide you to ensure that your hair and skin tones will flatter each other. For example, if you have gray hair and you want to go blonde, you won't be able to cover the gray. Blonding will just enhance the hair and make it look lighter, which will serve as excellent camouflage. As you get older, you don't want your hair color to be too dark either, because your gray regrowth will show up within two weeks. Plus, super-dark hair can be too harsh for more mature complexions.

HAIRDRESSER

One of the best ways to find the right hairdresser is to look for people with your hair type and great-looking hair. This is usually a good sign that their hairdresser will know how to cut and style your hair too. Even if it's a stranger on the street, just march right up to her and ask who does her hair. Believe me, no one will be insulted if you tell her that her hair looks great—you'll probably even make her day.

Price matters

The quality of hair care is related to price, but only to a degree. One hairdresser may be much more talented than another who charges the same price. If you live in a larger city, read reviews of top salons and hairdressers in style magazines and newspapers.

A good hairdresser will give you a great haircut you can work with. Also, master stylists often train their assistants or younger staff to cut, style, or color the way they do, but the assistant's services will be a lot more affordable. Just ask.

Talk about specialties

Every hairdresser has different talents and abilities. Some only cut hair, some just do color and chemical work, while others (like me) do it all. It makes no difference whether your stylist handles all aspects of your hair needs or whether you use professionals who specialize in each step—as long as you are pleased with the results.

But do find a stylist who specializes in your hair type. For example, if you have curly hair, make sure you find someone who styles and cuts curly hair well.

Time for a change

Some stylists will automatically update your look over time, which is great. Others get stuck in a rut—giving you the same look year after year. If you've asked your hairdresser for an updated look, but he or she still isn't giving you what you want, you might want to try someone else. It's not a crime to experiment with different stylists. Don't let guilt keep you from making a change.

Testing the waters

A lot of hairdressers offer consultations. But, you can't really know how someone works and behaves until you experience it for yourself. Before taking the plunge for a haircut or a whole new style makeover, I think it's a far better idea to book a blow-dry. You'll learn a lot about how he or she handles hair in general and your hair in particular. You can discuss your hair as it's being worked on, and you can see if you feel comfortable with the stylist. Don't be afraid to do research, visit lots of different hairdressers in different salons, and test each with a blow-dry. Make it a project and have fun with it.

If you're preparing for your wedding and are going to be wearing an updo, you'll want to do test runs like this several months before the big day. Book updos at salons around the city so you can find one that's absolutely perfect. Please don't leave this until the last minute during this high-stress time. When you find a style you like, take a picture, and bring that for reference the day of the wedding.

Communication is key

Look for a hairdresser who is going to communicate with you. The number-one rule is, don't be afraid to ask questions. Good hairdressers will make recommendations. At the same time they'll listen to you and incorporate your requests, taking into consideration your taste and lifestyle. It's all give and take, but don't forget that communication works both ways. A hairdresser may be terrific but probably isn't psychic.

Get the picture

I'm never offended if a client brings in a photo of a style she loves, because it gives me a good idea of her taste. However, you must be realistic. Think of the photo as a guide rather than an absolute, and you'll be on the right track.

Your comfort level

Choosing a stylist and a salon is all about what makes you feel comfortable. If you like trendy, fashion-forward styling, look for a hairdresser who does that. If you like more classic, refined work, look for that. Some hairdressers are very loving and nurturing and will make you feel pampered. And there are other ones who don't have the time for all that but still do a great job. The kind you choose depends on how you feel and your taste.

products and tools

Good hair products and proper styling tools are the backbone of hairstyling. Even before you learn any styling techniques, you have to choose the products and tools that will work best for your hair.

There are as many different kinds of products and tools as there are hairstyles. The choices are endless, and the array can be confusing. But any hairdresser worth his or her salt narrows the seemingly infinite number of available options down to a few favorites they find work best. This is what I have done for you.

Please remember, what I suggest here are the products and tools that I have found to achieve the best results on the greatest number of people. This doesn't mean that if you find you get a better look with something else, you can't use and enjoy it. Without question, there are other products on the market that can be beneficial and work effectively. Use them! Ultimately, the choice is yours.

Hair products

The main things you need to know when choosing your hair products are:

- The products you choose *do* matter. If you use less expensive products, you run the risk of drying out your hair. If your hair is chemically treated (with hair color, relaxer, or perm), you even run the risk of stripping it and compounding the damage. Plus, most inexpensive products may have a higher percentage of water. You have to use more product to get results, which means that they can actually end up costing you more than professional-quality products do.

- Quality products don't weigh down the hair or create buildup. This means shorter drying time and less stress on the hair.

- Using the appropriate products not just for your hair type, but for your hair's condition at any particular time, is most effective. For example, if you have a gummy buildup from styling products, it is a good idea to wash your hair with a clarifying shampoo.

- It's always smart to use hair products with sunscreens (which also moisturize), particularly if you have color-treated or chemically processed hair, which is more delicate than untreated hair.

- Where styling products are concerned, less is more. A lot of people use too much styling product on their hair, which weighs down the hair, dirties it more quickly, and perhaps even causes an itchy, flaky scalp if the product was applied directly to the scalp.

- A clean scalp is the first step to a beautiful style. When shampooing and conditioning, you have to wash and massage your head in warm water and rinse thoroughly in cool water, or your hair and scalp won't be clean. And if they aren't clean, your hair won't be shiny and you won't be able to create the hairstyle you want. Plus, over time you'll risk having a gummy, flaky buildup.

- Real dandruff (compared to a flaky scalp from product buildup) or a skin condition such as psoriasis or eczema may not respond to dandruff shampoos. Consult your doctor or dermatologist for product recommendations.

Basic cleaning and conditioning products

Shampoo

Cleans the hair and the scalp. To keep hair clean and healthy, shampoo one to three times a week.

CLARIFYING SHAMPOO Deep-cleaning formula for removing styling product buildup.

MOISTURIZING SHAMPOO Helps restore moisture to hair. Also known as shampoo for dry, damaged, colored, or chemically treated hair.

DANDRUFF SHAMPOO Keeps flakes to a minimum.

Conditioner

Adds shine, body, softness, smoothness, and pliability to your hair after shampooing.

MOISTURIZING CONDITIONER Helps restore moisture to hair. Also known as conditioner for dry, damaged, colored, or chemically treated hair.

DETANGLER Removes difficult knots and tangles after shampooing and conditioning. Using a leave-in detangler is optional but is especially good for children's hair.

SHINE PRODUCT The one true essential for everyone to use on wet hair in preparation for styling to smooth, soften, give a glasslike sheen, and protect against the heat of the blow dryer. Also great to combat static electricity and humidity.

GLOSS A once-a-month treatment to enhance shine and protect colored hair.

Styling products

The function of all styling products is to change the texture of the hair so that it styles more easily and to give it the appearance of more density, thickness, and shine. Remember, when it comes to any product, less is always more. **For information on applying these products**, see pages 64–65.

Gel

Adds volume, calms down frizz, and makes hair feel thicker. Use for a quick slicked-back look on all hair types or to lock in curl on wavy or curly hair without frizz. Apply before or after styling, setting, or blow-drying.

REGULAR Medium hold for a slicked-back look, for locking in curl, and for calming frizz. Comes in a squeeze tube or pump.

SPRAY The same hold as regular gel but for those who don't want to get the product on their hands. Use to add volume before drying, or to set a style after drying.

SCULPTING Heavier, thicker formula for an extra-strong hold.

Pomade

Takes away fullness for a flatter, sleeker look. Straightens hair, locks in a style, and eliminates frizz. Removes surface frizzies.

STICK Locks out surface pouf and frizz.

STRAIGHTENING Takes the frizz out of hair and adds weight to curly or kinky hair to keep it from swelling and getting big.

Mousse

Pumps up and holds superfine or limp hair. Use to create lift and volume. On wet hair, mousse is great for helping to lock in curl on naturally curly hair and roller sets.

Finishing products

The role of finishing products is to create a polished look. They smooth out fly-aways and hold hair in place for longer-lasting styles.

Hairspray

Holds hair during finishing and afterward. The best hairsprays do <u>not contain</u> <u>lacquer</u> (which builds up into a sticky, resistant film that is nearly impossible to remove).

PUMP Holds but still allows some movement.

AEROSOL A fine mist locks in a hairstyle for fine hair. Is available in regular or extra-hold formulas.

Volumizing products

The (literally) biggest news in hair-care products is volumizing products. There is a whole subcategory of products devoted to adding volume to the hair. They work by puffing up the hair and giving the appearance that you have more hair or thicker hair than you actually do.

Volumizing products are a lifesaver for thin or limp hair (sometimes known as Chihuahua hair, cat hair, or angel hair) because of the lift and body they provide. I also have clients with thick hair who use volumizing products to lift some of the heavy look out of their hair.

Volumizing products cover the gamut and duplicate the function of products for regular hair. They include shampoo, conditioner, hairspray, and gel. Volumizing mist is the one product that is unique to the category. Always use volumizing mist and volumizing gel in combination on damp hair after shampooing and before drying to add a feeling of texture, body, fullness, and lift. They're also great for men concerned with thinning hair. Remember, less is more. A small amount of a volumizing product goes a long way.

Tools

In this book you'll notice that the predominant heat-styling tool I use is the blow dryer. This is because the blow dryer (and occasionally the hood dryer) is the only heat-styling tool I advocate for the nonprofessional with straight, wavy, or curly hair. In my salon it's what I use 95 percent of the time to style my clients' hair. After blow-drying hair, those with particularly stubborn kinky hair must also use a flattening iron to get their hair under control. Using the flattening iron takes some practice to master and must be done with care.

I have heard too many horror stories (thousands if you add them up) from both home users and professional hairdressers about the damage that electric rollers and curling irons can do to hair. With heat-styling tools the damage is a one-way street; once you've burned your hair, there's very little you can do to salvage it, other than to cut off the burned ends.

If you use the styling techniques I have developed over the years and share with you now, the blow dryer (along with the proper products, of course) can do absolutely everything for you that other heat-styling instruments can do. I promise you that with a little practice, you'll be able to achieve any look you want—and in the same amount of time. Wait, I'll up the stakes here a little—let's make it any look you want in even less time. **For more on the basics of caring for your hair, see pages 54–67, and to learn how to create beautiful, finished styles, see pages 68–159.**

Dryers and accessories

Blow dryer

USE To dry and style hair.

LOOK FOR 1600 watts or higher. Remember, the higher the wattage, the greater the heat, the less time it takes to dry the hair, and the less long-term stress on the hair. Look for a blow dryer that is not too heavy and is comfortable for you to hold and maneuver.

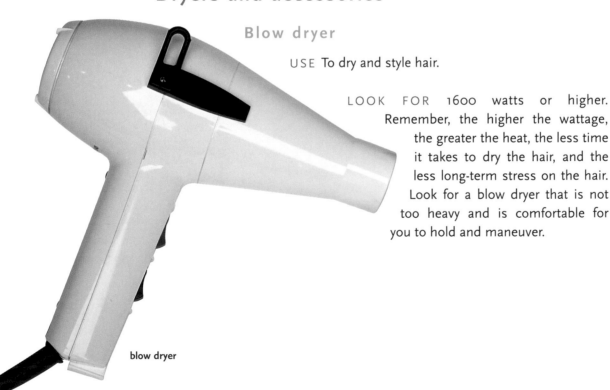

blow dryer

Air-compressor nozzle

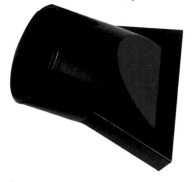

USE To get hair poker straight and flat and remove the volume.

LOOK FOR A blow dryer that comes with one (most do).

Diffuser sock

USE To control the direction of the heat on the blow dryer, minimize frizz, lock in curl, lock in a style more quickly, and create fullness.

LOOK FOR A synthetic, elastic one-size-fits-all sock (a.k.a. diffuser mitt) that fits over the blow dryer head. There are also large disc-shaped collar units available, but I think they're too large and cumbersome.

Hood dryer

USE To dry hair over roller sets.

LOOK FOR Multiple heat controls and a hood that feels comfortable on your head.

diffuser sock

Flattening iron

USE To get kinky hair sleek and smooth after setting and drying. Great for bangs and removing frizz from kinky hair too.

LOOK FOR A hinged clamp that feels comfortable in your hand and isn't too heavy.

flattening iron

Brushes

Round brush with perforated metal cylinder

USE To use with the blow dryer to encourage lift, volume, and smooth hair. The perforated metal cylinder heats up to lock in the curl or wave. Used with the blow dryer, the perforated metal cylinder also saves drying time (and hair stress) because it enables you to dry both sides of the hair simultaneously. However, it is very important to insert a stick-on roller while the hair is still warm, immediately after blowing each section dry with the heated brush (this locks in curl and volume).

LOOK FOR Medium size, metal cylinder perforated by holes, and pliable bristles. Once you master the medium-size brush, you can experiment with other sizes to suit your taste and style.

Wooden styling brush

USE To brush, finish, smooth, and detangle dry hair.

LOOK FOR A brush that feels good in the hand; movable, pliable bristles.

round brush
with perforated metal cylinder

wooden styling brush

Combs

Wide-tooth comb

USE To comb the hair free of tangles when wet or dry. Also great for back-combing to create a more natural look.

LOOK FOR A comb that feels good in the hand; plastic, with smooth edges.

Rat-tail (teasing) comb

USE To section precisely, back-comb, and style. The tail on the comb is good for lifting hair for volume or lift.

LOOK FOR A comb that feels good in the hand. Remember, the smaller the teeth, the tighter the tease and the wider the teeth, the more natural the tease.

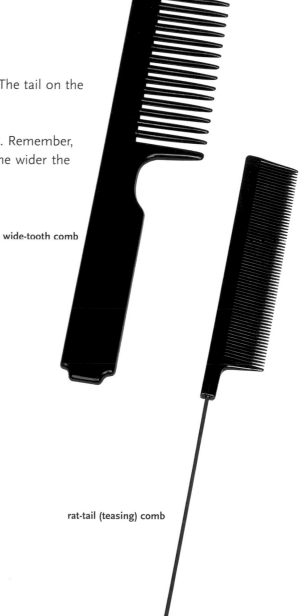

wide-tooth comb

rat-tail (teasing) comb

Setting and holding

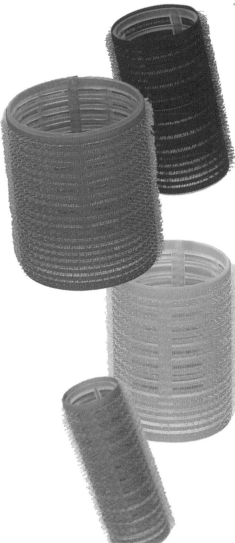

Stick-on rollers

USE To create lift, volume, smooth hair, or curls after a blow-dry; for a dry roller set to refresh a hairstyle or a wet set under the dryer. Even if you're all thumbs, these are simple to use to get a great look.

LOOK FOR An assortment of different sizes for different effects (the smaller the roller, the tighter the curl).

Large clips

USE To hold sections or rollers, to create waves and quick sets without rollers, or to anchor an updo.

LOOK FOR Those at least 4 inches in length.

Bobby pins

USE To hold flatter styles or anchor an updo.

LOOK FOR Regular and large sizes in a color to match your hair, with rubber tips. Remember never to use your teeth to open bobby pins.

Hairpins

USE To hold updos.

LOOK FOR Various sizes, weights, and colors.

Covered elastic bands

USE To secure ponytails or braids on dry hair. Regular rubber bands can pull and break the hair off.

Spray bottle

USE To spritz water on a section of hair if it dries before you have a chance to style it. Good to lightly mist curly hair if it falls flat.

LOOK FOR A bottle that spritzes a fine mist, not big drops.

Plastic shower cap

USE To cover hair for conditioning treatments or to save your hairstyle as you shower.

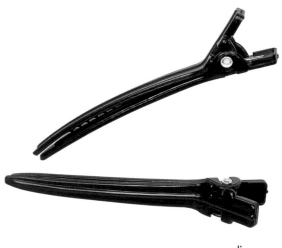

clips

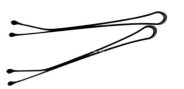

bobby pins

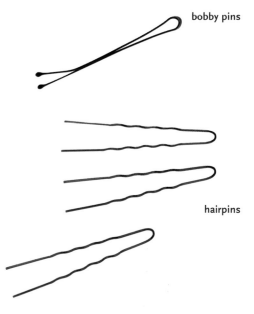

hairpins

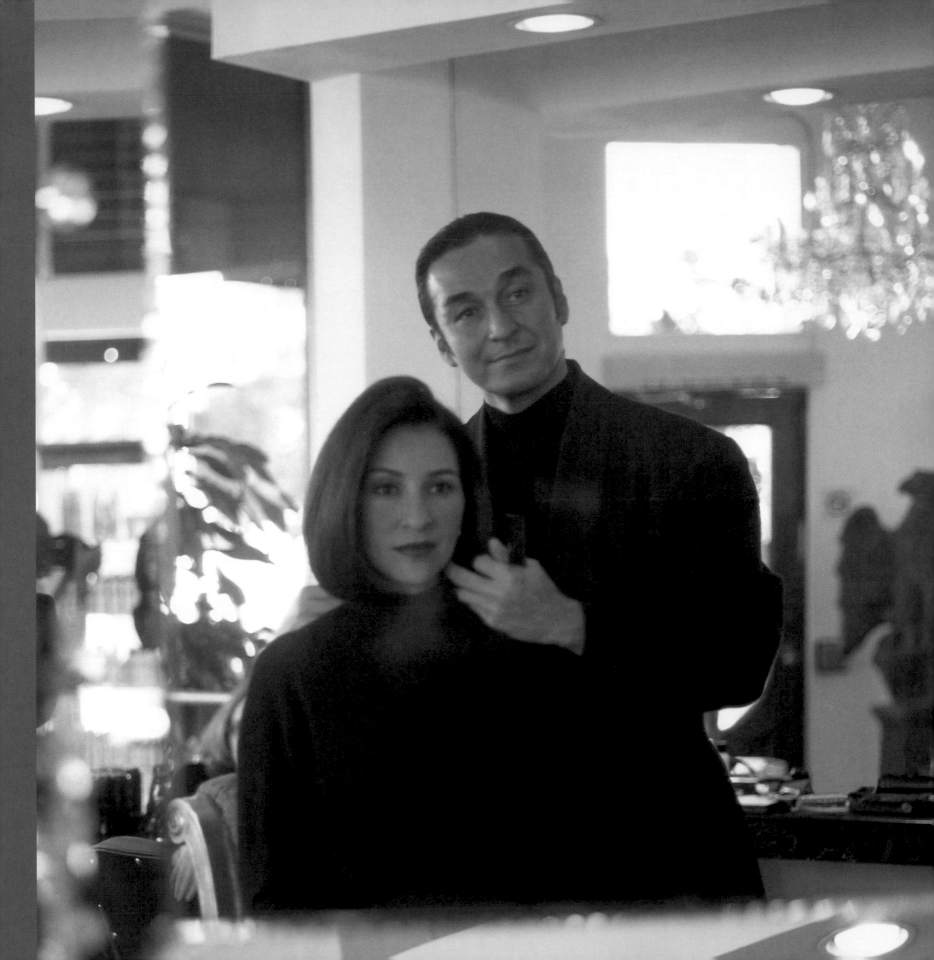

THE BASICS

2

cleaning and care basics

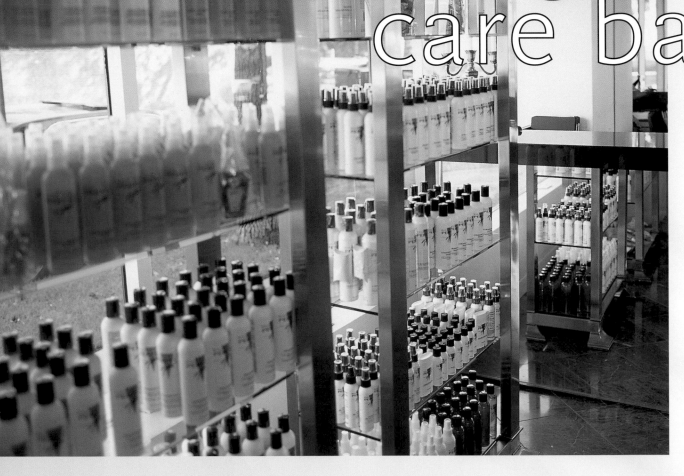

You may think you already know how to wash your hair. Or you may feel that there's nothing more you need to know about brushing it. Or you may think you've got styling products down pat. Well, maybe so, maybe not.

This chapter may seem elementary, but I urge you to review it carefully. I can't tell you how many people I hear complain about hair problems, convinced that there's something terribly wrong, when in fact the "problem" is that they're just not taking care of their hair correctly. Here are some of the most common mistakes people make when caring for their hair . . . and the results.

Washing and drying too often = Potential damage

We shampoo our hair too frequently. Washing your hair too often (particularly when accompanied by heat-styling and drying) can leave it dry, limp, damaged, and bushy by robbing it of its natural oils and luster. Unless you have an extremely oily scalp, a skin condition, or regularly subject your hair to a harsh environment (cigarette smoke, chlorinated pool water, and the like), you should not wash it daily. And once you learn to style it properly, you won't want to because your hair will look beautiful for days. In fact, your hair will usually look better on the second day. An added bonus: Since you're not washing your hair as frequently, you'll save money on products and plenty of time.

Improper rinsing = Residue and flaking

Not rinsing your hair properly and thoroughly can leave it difficult to manage and looking dull and lifeless. Over time, product residue can result in a dry, flaky, and itchy scalp or for those with an oily scalp, a greasy, irritated, itchy, and flaky scalp.

Improper heat-styling = Potential damage

Too much or the wrong kind of heat-styling with dryers, curling irons, electric rollers, and other implements can burn, break, and damage your hair.

Too much product = Dirt and unmanageability

Using too much of a product on your scalp or hair—whether it be a conditioning or styling product—makes the hair dirty, weighs it down, and makes it look dull. Residue and buildup result in hair and scalp problems.

The wrong shampoo = Dry hair

Washing with shampoo that is too harsh for your hair can dry it out or strip colored hair.

Rough treatment when wet = Potential damage

Handling your hair improperly while it is wet can cause breakage, split ends, and even hair loss.

Washing without clarifying = Scummy buildup

Not using a clarifying shampoo at least occasionally (particularly if you use a lot of styling products) means that scalp problems, unattractive product residue, and irritation are with you to stay.

Repairing your hair

You can repair your hair with the right products. But if your hair has split ends, the best thing to do is to bite the bullet and trim it. It's that simple.

Meanwhile, as you grow healthy hair, good products can provide something of a bandage effect. Eventually, if you keep using the proper products, washing your hair and scalp correctly, heat-styling it correctly, and letting it air-dry occasionally, you will notice that your hair feels and looks healthier. The improvement will be gradual, but it will be real.

Of course, not all your hair and scalp problems will disappear if you put into practice the suggestions that follow. But work these practices into your routine and you'll be delighted with the instant benefits.

SHAMPOO AND CONDITION YOUR HAIR

1 Before getting your hair wet, first remove any tangles or knots with a comb or soft-bristle brush, starting at the ends and working your way up toward the scalp.

2 Wet your hair thoroughly with warm water.

3 Pour a dollop of shampoo about the size of a quarter into your hand, then rub your palms together once or twice (never put a blob of shampoo directly onto your hair or scalp).

4 Using your fingertips, thoroughly massage the shampoo (which will begin to become sudsy) evenly into your scalp. Massage each section of your head for about a minute. Don't rush; the more you massage your scalp, the better you clean it and the more you stimulate blood circulation there.

5 Rinse with cool water (it doesn't have to be cold). Most people do not rinse thoroughly enough, which results in scummy buildup. Be sure to let the water hit your head for about a minute at every angle. You may find it helpful to rake your fingers through your hair and lift it up by the roots to get more water closer to your scalp.

6 If you need a second shampoo, repeat Steps 3–5. How do you tell? If your shampoo gets really sudsy during your first lather, you hair is clean enough already. If not, shampoo a second time—there's still grime that needs to be shampooed away.

7 Gently squeeze excess water out of your hair.

8 Put a quarter-size dollop of conditioner in the palm of one hand and rub your palms together.

9 Apply the conditioner to your hair only, working it up from the ends and keeping it at least 2 inches away from the scalp. Applying conditioner to

your scalp will cause it to get oily and greasy sooner than it should. If you have fine, limp hair or long hair in good condition, you can get away with conditioning only the ends or stopping 2 to 3 inches away from the scalp. (If you use a leave-in conditioner, stop here. If you use the rinse-out kind, continue on to Steps 10 and 11.)

10 Leave the conditioner in for a minute or two (or if you're in the shower, for as long as it takes you to wash the rest of your body) before rinsing.

11 Rinse thoroughly with cool water.

This icon is used throughout the book to refer back to these instructions for shampooing and conditioning your hair.

notes on

SHAMPOOING AND CONDITIONING LONG HAIR

If you have long hair, shampooing and conditioning it in the shower is the best bet because the water can do some of the work for you. Follow the instructions above, and be sure to brush or comb your hair before you shower. This will save a lot of potential breakage when your hair is wet later.

As you wet your head, let the warm water run down the length of your hair and down your back. Be careful not to mash the shampoo into your hair in one big glob or it will cause the hair to mat. Use your fingertips to massage the scalp only with gentle circular movements. Big circular movements will cause all kinds of tangles and knots in your hair.

Condition as directed above and rinse with cool water, letting it pour straight down over your hair (which will help the detangling process a lot). At the same time you may want to run a wide-tooth comb or soft-bristle brush through your hair (again, always from the ends up until the tangles or knots are gone) as the water cascades down. The rule of thumb to remember is always shampoo the scalp, condition the hair. If you use a leave-in conditioner, skip Steps 10 and 11.

DEEP-CONDITION OR MOISTURIZE YOUR HAIR

Some people feel that they need a little extra conditioning from time to time (if your hair feels like a haystack, it's a pretty good sign that you do too). One easy trick is to turn your regular conditioner into a moisture pack at home. You can do this once a week if necessary. You shouldn't do it more than that, though, or you risk causing a sticky, heavy, and oily buildup.

QUICK-FIX MOISTURE PACK After shampooing and rinsing, apply the conditioner as usual, taking care to keep it away from the roots. Instead of rinsing after a minute or two, wrap your head in a towel or plastic bag and leave the conditioner in your hair for about 15 minutes before rinsing with cool water.

TOWEL DRY YOUR HAIR

Wet hair is vulnerable hair. If you grab all of your hair when it's wet and twist it tight, you'll snap some strands of hair right off. If you rub your wet head back and forth too vigorously with a towel, you'll actually break the hair and may even cause split ends. Instead of towel-drying, think of it as *towel-blotting*, and you'll be on the right track.

TOWEL-DRYING SHORT TO MEDIUM-LENGTH HAIR Use the palms of your hands like a squeegee to extract as much wetness as possible. Then scrunch your hair very lightly with your fingers to squeeze out as much water as can easily be removed. Then—and only then—press the towel into the hair to blot away moisture.

TOWEL-DRYING LONG HAIR While you're still in the shower, glide your hands down the length of your hair to rid it of the excess water. Then press the towel into your hair to blot excess water from it.

drying tip

GIVE STRAIGHT AND WAVY HAIR A BREAK FROM THE HEAT Taking your hair from sopping wet to bone dry can be pretty traumatic for it if you always use heat. If you have the time—even if it's only 5 or 10 minutes—let your hair air-dry until it is damp before taking the blow dryer to it. You'll still be able to get all the styling versatility you need, and you will put a lot less stress on your hair. Over time, your hair will be healthier for it. (Curly and kinky hair types, on the other hand, need heat-styling immediately to curb frizz and to get the hair to behave properly.)

how to

UNTANGLE AND COMB WET HAIR

To protect your hair, there are a few things you should remember when combing it:

- Always detangle from the ends and work up to the scalp.

- Use small, slow strokes with a wide-tooth comb. You risk snapping off the hair if you use big, quick ones.

- Always start combing from about an inch or two above the ends. When that section of the hair is smooth, move up an inch or two and continue combing down until the new area is also smooth. Proceed in this way, moving up inch by inch, until you've worked your way to the scalp.

COMBING SHORT TO MEDIUM-LENGTH HAIR Moving from the ends to the scalp, start at the nape of your neck, work up to the crown of your head, comb the front, and finish with the sides. Comb straight back from the forehead in preparation for styling.

COMBING MEDIUM-LENGTH TO LONG HAIR First gather your hair together in a ponytail with your hand and start combing from the bottom to remove any knots or tangles from the ends. Release the hair and, in increments, starting at the ends on the nape of your neck, work your way up from the bottom to the crown, then to the front and the sides, until your hair is perfectly smooth before combing from scalp to ends. If your hair is very thick, it may be easier to section and clip it first and then comb out each section individually.

BRUSH DRY HAIR

There are two schools of thought on brushing hair. Some say it's great to brush hair frequently because brushing distributes the hair's natural oils along the entire length of the hair shaft; others say it's not good because it overstimulates the scalp and can aggravate hair loss. Personally, I like brushing because I think it lends a nice sheen to the hair. But in my opinion, whether you brush or not is entirely up to you. If you enjoy brushing your hair, do it and savor the great feeling. But if you don't enjoy it, don't feel you need to do it.

To protect your hair and ensure the health of your scalp, however, there are a few things you should remember when you do brush your hair. Many of the same rules apply for using a brush as for using a comb:

- Use small, slow strokes with a wooden styling brush. You risk snapping off the hair if you use big, quick ones.

- Always start brushing from about an inch or two above the ends. When that section of the hair is smooth, move up an inch or two and continue brushing down until the new area is also smooth. Proceed in this way, moving up inch by inch, until you've worked your way to the scalp.

- If your hair is tangled, comb it first. Never, ever brush your hair from the scalp to the ends if it has any tangles. From the bottom, work the tangles out first with a wide-tooth comb, then brush. Or if you have really bad tangles and knots, put a drop of shine product onto your hair (when wet or dry) and then pick the hair apart very slowly from bottom to top.

- If your hair is newly clean, overenthusiastic brushing may cause it to snap off. It is best to postpone brushing after washing so that your hair can generate some natural oils.

- If you have a flaky scalp, a gentle scalp massage along with brushing may help to dislodge the flakes. (If, however, you have psoriasis or another skin problem on your scalp, brushing may scratch the skin and irritate it.)

BRUSHING SHORT TO MEDIUM-LENGTH HAIR In increments, start at the ends on the nape of your neck, work up to the crown, brush the sides, and finish with the front. When your hair is perfectly tangle free, you can then brush from scalp to ends.

BRUSHING MEDIUM-LENGTH TO LONG HAIR First gather your hair together in a ponytail with your hand and start brushing from the bottom to remove any knots or tangles from the ends. Release the hair and, in increments, starting at the ends on the nape of your neck, always brushing down, work your way up from the bottom to the crown, then to the front and the sides, until your hair is perfectly smooth before brushing from scalp to ends. If your hair is very thick, it may be easier to section and clip it first and then brush out each section individually.

notes on LONG HAIR

In the old days, when a girl got married, she was expected to cut her hair. Even in our lifetime a woman of a certain age (it used to be thirty a generation ago; today it's about forty) is expected to cut her hair. Personally, I love long hair, and I believe that you don't have to cut it if you don't want to. If you like your long hair and you feel good about it, then you should keep it. Don't worry about what anybody else says. The most important thing is that you feel comfortable with yourself.

The only thing that matters to me—and it matters a lot—is that, if you're going to wear long hair, make sure you have great long hair. That means your hair has lots of shine, isn't broken off, and the ends are trimmed regularly.

Long hair requires a little extra attention because it's been around longer and has had more time to get damaged. People with long hair have to be careful not to pull it too hard, bind it too tightly, or braid it too tight (or wear it in an elastic band at night, which will snap hairs right off, I guarantee). Be gentle. Long hair is to be enjoyed, not punished. Throughout this book I've noted special techniques for long hair wearers.

APPLY STYLING PRODUCTS ON WET HAIR

On the one hand, you don't want to use too much product. On the other, remember that you're styling in three dimensions and you want all of your hair to look good, not just the parts you can see in the mirror. Don't just plop product on top of your hair; make sure you work it into the hair evenly.

Shine product

FOR WHAT AND WHEN To add strength, flexibility, resilience, and shine. Use on wet hair right after towel-drying and before or after styling.

HOW MUCH TO USE 1 to 3 pea-size drops, depending on the thickness of your hair.

HOW TO APPLY Put the product on your hands first, rub your palms together, then rub your hands through your hair from back to front. Make sure to cover the ends too.

CAUTIONARY NOTE Do not use too much product or use it on the roots because it can weigh the roots down and make your hair appear dirty. Apply it to the ends first.

Straightening pomade

FOR WHAT AND WHEN To straighten or to hold before or after styling, setting, or blow-drying. To take the pouf out of hair for a sleeker, straighter look.

HOW MUCH TO USE Depending on hair type, style, and length, start with a dollop the size of a dime.

HOW TO APPLY Put the product on your hands first, rub your palms together, then rub your hands through your hair from back to front.

CAUTIONARY NOTE Do not use any oily or waxy pomades on the roots because they can weigh the roots down and make your hair appear dirty.

Gel and mousse

FOR WHAT AND WHEN To create lift and volume. On wet hair, gel and mousse are great for helping to lock in curl.

HOW MUCH TO USE Depending on hair type, style, and length, start with a dollop of gel the size of a dime or a dollop of mousse the size of a golf ball, then add more as needed.

HOW TO APPLY Put the product on your hands first, rub your palms together, then rub your hands through your hair from back to front.

CAUTIONARY NOTE Don't use gel on the roots because it can weigh them down and make your hair look dirty. Don't be fooled by mousse's light, airy texture. It can get very sticky and cause buildup if you use too much.

Spritzes and spray gel

FOR WHAT AND WHEN To create volume before drying.

HOW MUCH TO USE Start with one spritz per section. Apply more as needed.

HOW TO APPLY Spritz from about 1 inch away for extra volume at the roots.

how to APPLY HAIRSPRAY

FOR WHAT AND WHEN Holds hair during finishing and afterward.

HOW MUCH TO USE Depending on hair type, style, and length, start with a single spritz per section, or in case of the whole head, 3 to 5 spritzes.

HOW TO APPLY Always apply hairspray from 10 to 12 inches above the area you're targeting, spritz, and then let the spray gently mist down onto the hair.

CAUTIONARY NOTE Use a hairspray that does not contain lacquer (which builds up into a sticky, resistant film that is nearly impossible to remove).

Preventing and treating environmental damage

It is a lot easier to prevent the effects of a harsh environment than to repair the damage it causes to your hair after the fact.

Sun

LOOKS LIKE Bleached-out color; dry, strawlike texture.

PREVENTION For regular daily activities, you can protect your hair by using conditioning and styling products with UVA sunscreens. If you're going to be outdoors for an extended period or if you're sitting in the sun, your hair needs extra moisture and protection. Work a generous amount of conditioner through your hair (wet or dry) before you go outside, or work the sunscreen you use on your skin into your hair—don't worry, the grease will wash out easily. If you have long hair, conditioning and then braiding it can help protect it. The most sensible solution, of course, is to wear a hat.

TREATMENT Wash your hair with a moisturizing shampoo and leave the conditioner on for 20 minutes. Wrap your head in plastic wrap or put on a shower cap to encourage the conditioner to penetrate more deeply.

Air pollution and cigarette smoke

LOOKS LIKE A yellowish tinge on light or gray hair. Hair smells awful too.

PREVENTION Don't smoke. I know it's hard, but don't do it.

TREATMENT Wash hair with a clarifying shampoo and condition thoroughly.

Chlorine

LOOKS LIKE Increased porosity and brittleness; a green tinge on blonde and light-colored hair, discoloration in other hair colors. When the sun bakes chlorine into hair, the damage multiplies. Hair loses body and shine and breaks off easily.

PREVENTION Work conditioner (or a silicone product such as a shine) into your hair to protect it before you go into the water. If possible, also wear a swim cap while spending any time in chlorinated water.

TREATMENT After swimming, wash your hair immediately with a clarifying shampoo and condition thoroughly. Never let chlorine dry in your hair.

Saltwater

LOOKS LIKE Stripped color, discoloration, dryness, and increased porosity.

PREVENTION Work conditioner (or a silicone product such as a shine) into your hair to protect it before you go into the water. If possible, also wear a swim cap while spending any time in saltwater.

TREATMENT After swimming, wash your hair immediately with a clarifying shampoo and condition thoroughly. If you don't have access to a shower, you can rinse your hair with club soda or mineral water to neutralize the salt.

Hard water

LOOKS LIKE Dry, brittle texture.

PREVENTION Install a water filter in your home.

TREATMENT Wash your hair with a clarifying shampoo and leave the conditioner on for 20 minutes. To encourage the conditioner to penetrate more deeply, wrap your head in plastic wrap or put on a shower cap. Use a shine product before styling.

Cold weather

LOOKS LIKE Flyaway, caused by static electricity. Going from a hot room into the cold outdoors dries out your hair and causes the static electricity.

PREVENTION AND TREATMENT Wash your hair with a moisturizing shampoo, condition thoroughly, and use a shine product before styling.

styling basics

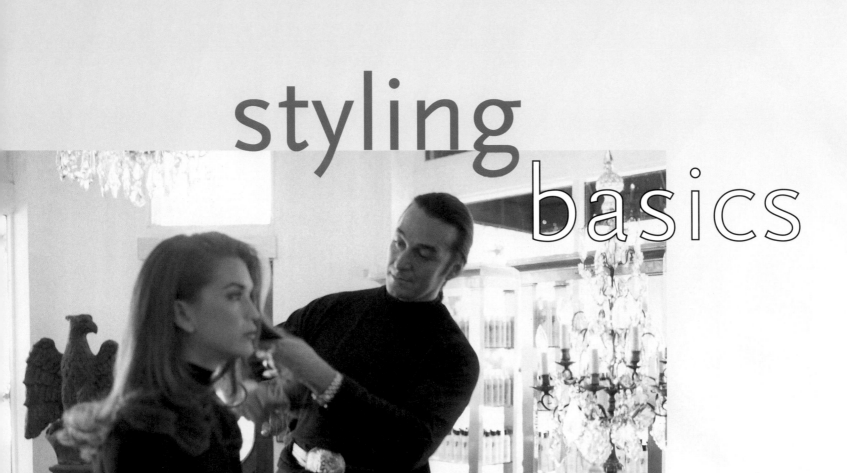

Many women tell me that when they walk out of a salon after they have their hair cut and styled, they're happy and in love with their hair. But the minute they wash their hair at home and try to duplicate the look themselves, they say, "Oh no, it's not the same!" It's not unreasonable to want a pretty, polished, frizz-free, and finished look with shine and manageability that you can reproduce by yourself, is it? It shouldn't be so hard to get—right? It won't be with just a few basic techniques under your belt.

I want to emphasize that the steps I'm describing here are methods that I have found to work for my clients and for me. You may find that you achieve results using some other method, or as you go through this book, you may come up with some shortcuts to get the look you want. To all of that I say great and go for it. Let's get to work.

For those who have been unhappy with home hairstyling, what I'm offering here is a step-by-step guide that explains how to turn a frustrating experience into an easy, time-saving, enjoyable one—with beautiful results. I want you to use this information as you would the recipes in a cookbook; take what you need, adapt it to your talents and taste, and make it your own.

The biggest styling and blow-drying mistakes I see happen when people try to rush the process and end up blowing frizz and tangles into their hair or inadvertently blowing volume out of their hair. Or they hold the dryer in one place for too long and end up burning their hair. Or they use way too much product, which weighs down their hair and makes it dirty, limp, and impossible to style. Or they pull on the brush so hard while blow-drying that they end up pulling out their hair by the roots or breaking it off.

The secret to successful, professional-looking styling is to slow down, get organized, don't panic, and don't forget to use both hands if you need to.

For most of the styling and blow-drying that I do and am showing you here, the key is to do it step-by-step, one section at a time. We'll start with learning how to section, the backbone to professional hairdressing, and then move forward to the basic blow-dry.

Hairstyling is all about creating a frame for your picture . . . you. In the beginning, if tackling your whole head seems overwhelming, don't worry. Essentially, you'll be doing your hair one section at a time, getting it right, and then moving on to the next section. Before you know it, you'll be done. And gorgeous.

All about sectioning

Learning to section will change your approach to hairstyling forever and give you enormous confidence. Sectioning is what differentiates professional hairdressers from most nonprofessionals. But it's not all that difficult, and I guarantee that if you master this, the rest is a breeze.

Basically, sectioning is parting the hair all over the head into different areas and clipping each section out of the way except for the one you're working on. Different hair professionals section hair in slightly different configurations, but I've found that a standardized six sections, with each location labeled by number, works best on short or long hair (see pages 72–73).

Eventually, you may find that you don't need to section quite as diligently to get the look you like. I have no problem with that; shortcuts are always great

if they work for you. But in the beginning, take the time to learn sectioning, learn it well, and really understand it. Getting the hang of sectioning is like learning to master anything.

You can section with a comb or with your fingers. Usually we'll work with a wide-tooth comb. You can section hair when it is wet, damp, or dry. Most often, except in the case of a touch-up or an updo, we'll section the hair when it is towel-dried. You can secure sections with a hair clip or a bobby pin. For our purposes, large hair clips are the most effective to keep your hair from blowing all over and tangling up when you dry it.

The advantages of sectioning are numerous:

PROVIDES ORDER The most important thing to remember about sectioning is that it provides a system for keeping everything in sequence. It cues you which part of your hair to style first (that is, you'll always begin with Section 1: bangs/front) and in what order to proceed. By beginning with Section 1, you'll always start with the area that is most visible, gets the most attention, and is usually the trickiest.

ORGANIZES BLOW-DRYING If you have wavy, curly, or kinky hair, random blow-drying can turn your hair into a frizzy, unmanageable mess. By sectioning and blow-drying your hair a piece at a time, lock by lock, you'll get exactly the degree of smoothness and volume you desire, exactly where you want it, without messing up the rest of your hair. As soon as you blow-dry one section, you clip it up or put it in a roller to keep it out of the way (and to lock in the style) as you style subsequent sections.

LEADS TO OTHER SKILLS Once you master sectioning, styling techniques you may have thought were way out of your league suddenly become possible. Dry roller sets, wet sets, and updos will turn into simple exercises in logic. Learning to section will also teach you how to handle your hair properly—lifting up your arms to get the leverage you need to work with your hair (and it's great exercise for those arms too!).

SAVES TIME (AND YOUR SANITY) Hairdressing isn't a random exercise. Sectioning your hair, working on one piece at a time, and then securing it out of the way, is a real time-saver because you won't end up redoing the same section over and over again (which would damage your hair). Plus, you won't end up undoing the work you've already done.

Sectioning savvy

Knowing how to divide your hair into "The Big Six" sections gives you the basis for creating any hairstyle. When you style your hair, you'll almost always do it section by section, in numerical order. With practice, sectioning will become second nature.

Section 1: bangs/front

Your bangs. If you don't have bangs, Section 1 runs from temple to temple, approximately 2 to 3 inches back from the top of your forehead.

Section 2: top/crown

The rectangular section on the top of your head, between the left and right parts, which extends back from Section 1 to the part running between your ears.

Section 3: left side

On the left side below Sections 1 and 2, extending from the hairline back to the part between your ears.

Section 4: right side

On the right side below Sections 1 and 2, extending from the hairline back to the part between your ears.

Section 5: back left

On the back left side behind Sections 2 and 3 and to the left of the center part.

Section 6: back right

On the back right side behind Sections 2 and 4 and to the right of the center part.

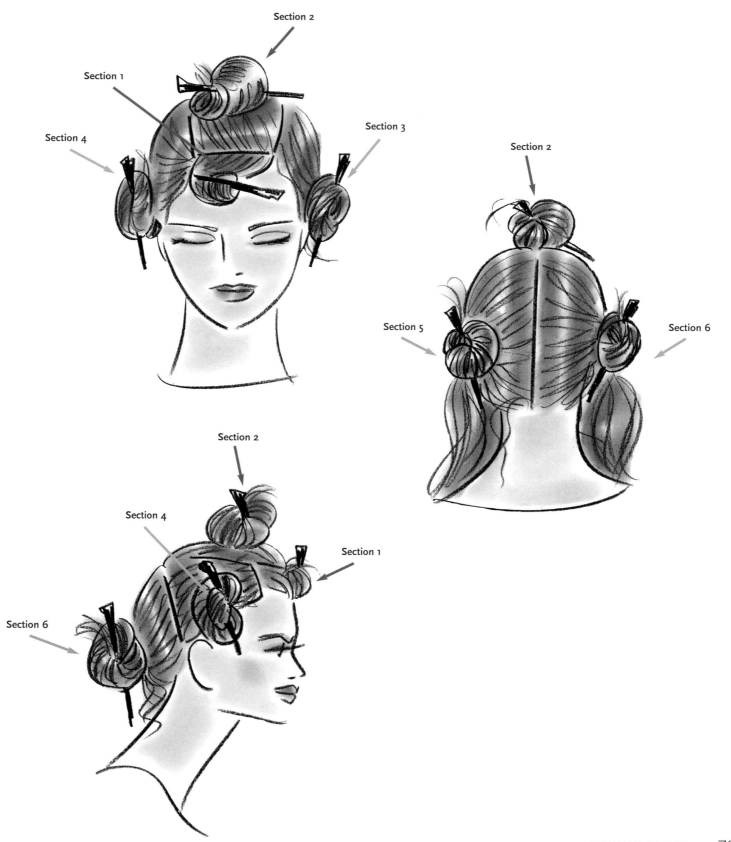

Section 2

Section 1

Section 4

Section 3

Section 2

Section 5

Section 6

Section 2

Section 4

Section 1

Section 6

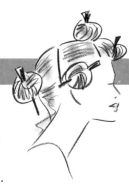

how to

SECTION YOUR HAIR

The Big Six (pages 72–73) represents the order in which you will work on your hair when styling it. Don't worry if your sections aren't exactly precise; your final hairstyle won't suffer. You don't have to create the sections in any particular order, but here's what works for me, step-by-step.

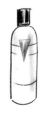

1   Shampoo, condition, and comb your damp or wet hair with a wide-tooth comb. Apply the first round of styling product. Whether you apply the product at the ends only or all over will depend on the kind of product and the style you are trying to achieve.

PAGE **58**

2   With your comb, run a part down the center of your head, from your forehead all the way back to the nape of your neck, dividing your hair along this part.

3   Create another part over the top of your head by running the comb from the hairline just behind one ear to the hairline just behind the other ear, so that now it looks like you have made a cross on the top of your head. (You'll have four big sections at this point.)

4   Create a part from your hairline at each temple back toward the part running from ear to ear made in the last step. If you have short hair, clip together the front/crown hair on each side of the center part. This area will later be parted from side to side to form Sections 1 and 2. If you have long hair, twist and clip this hair on top of your head.

5   Separately clip or twist and clip Sections 5 and 6 (back left and back right) to the back of your head, away from the back center part.

6   Over your left ear, clip or twist and clip Section 3 (left side). Over your right ear, clip or twist and clip Section 4 (right side).

7   Undo the clip at the top of your head and create a part across your head from temple to temple to separate Section 1 (bangs/front) from the top/crown of your head (Section 2). Clip or twist and clip Section 1.

8   Clip and twist Section 2 (top/crown).

 This icon is used throughout the book to refer to these instructions for sectioning your hair.

Drying and setting

After shampooing and conditioning your hair, there are really only three basic ways of taking your hair from wet to dry (and, we hope, adding some style to it in the process). You can let it air-dry, you can blow-dry it, or you can wet-set it and sit under a hood dryer. (Of course, you could wet-set it and sleep on the rollers overnight, but that's prehistoric torture as far as I'm concerned, and I know you really want your beauty sleep. Besides, it breaks your hair.)

Why air-drying will never equal high style

Every day I hear women tell me that they're too busy to blow-dry their hair, let alone put in stick-on rollers or anything else. Believe me, I understand, and nothing says that you can't just wash your hair and let it air-dry. Depending on your hair type, you can look pretty good.

If air-drying is the way you choose to go, either because of time constraints or your lifestyle, I urge you to get the very best haircut that you can because that haircut is going to be doing most of the work. (See pages 38–39 for some helpful hints on finding the right hairdresser and getting a great haircut.)

However—and this is where I get onto my soapbox—don't be fooled. With few exceptions, no matter how great the cut or how healthy your hair, if you let it air-dry, you can't expect to have a finished, salon-quality, professional look. Hair has to be styled and enhanced to look finished, particularly if you want volume and extra body.

Blow drying and keeping hair healthy

Maybe you're sensing a contradiction here. In Chapter 2 and Chapter 4, I go on and on about how blow dryers and improper heat-styling can thrash your hair and leave it damaged. Furthermore, I emphasize that shampooing less frequently is better for your hair and that air-drying when possible will improve its condition immeasurably. Now, I've just told you that air-drying won't give you the look you want. How can you win?

It's all a matter of degree. Using heat to go from soaking wet to bone dry is hard on your hair, true. That's why blotting your hair and towel-drying to remove as much water as possible after shampooing are so important. But here's the winning combination for most hair types (aside from kinky hair or curly hair that you want to make straight, straight, straight): if you apply the first round of styling product (shine) and let your hair air-dry partially until it is damp rather than wet, you'll cut your blow-drying time in half. You will eliminate an enormous amount of wear and tear from the heat, and even better, you'll still be able to achieve that polished look and every single one of the styling benefits you're looking for.

blow-dry tips

GO EASY ON THE STYLING PRODUCTS Depending on your hair type and style, the smallest amount of styling products is usually sufficient. Using any more may weigh down your hair and cause it to get so dirty you won't be able to blow-dry or style it properly. Start with less, then add more if you need to.

KEEP THE DRYER MOVING Holding the dryer in one place for too long can burn your scalp and damage your hair. Ouch!

volumizing tips

OVERDIRECT THE ROOTS FOR VOLUME Absolutely the most important component of creating volume, fullness, and lift in a style is to overdirect the roots. To overdirect, secure the ends of a hair section with a round brush or a roller set, and as you blow-dry it, hold the section up in the direction opposite to that in which you want it to lie.

Remember, overdirection affects how you direct the roots; it has nothing to do with what the ends of the hair will do. If you want the ends to roll under, while overdirecting the roots, place the brush under the ends, catch and wrap them, and roll the hair around the brush. If you want your ends to flip up, place the brush over the ends, catch and wrap them, and roll the hair around the brush.

WORK UP FROM UNDER FOR LIFT Working and directing the heat from underneath increases volume, as does flipping your head over at the beginning and using the blow dryer on a low-heat setting or with a diffuser to remove moisture.

GO EASY ON THE TENSION Don't pull too tight when you're holding a hair section on a round brush—save that for getting a super-straight look or for straightening curly hair. Use an especially light touch on thin hair.

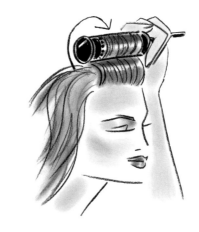

**overdirect roots,
Section 1**

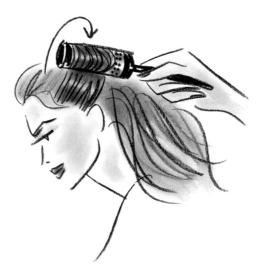

**overdirect roots,
Section 3**

How do I blow-dry? Let me count the ways . . .

We're going to spend a lot of time on step-by-step instructions for blow-drying your own hair because a professional salon look depends equally on the cut (which you probably don't do) and the blow-dry (which you'll be an expert on before we're through). By far and away the most efficient and popular way of simultaneously drying and styling your hair is with the blow dryer.

We refer to each of the following blow-dry methods throughout the book with the icons to the right. The different methods are:

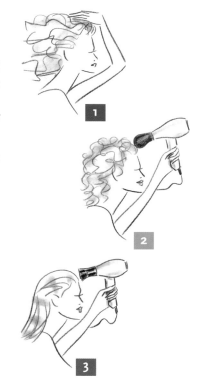

1 Blow-dry with fingers for a natural look.

2 Blow-dry with a diffuser to enhance curly hair.

3 Blow-dry smooth and straight.

4 Blow-dry with a round brush for volume.

5 Blow-dry with a round brush and rollers.

6 Wet-set for volume and extra hold.

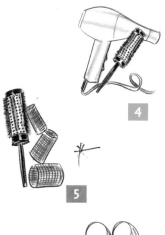

Some of these blow-drying techniques work better with different hair types than others, and not all of them require sectioning. With a little experimentation you'll find the one (or ones) that suit you best.

The majority of my clients—and we're talking about 90 percent here—ask for lots of volume, shine, body, and lift. Even those who crave shiny, straight hair still want it to have plenty of body and bounce. And everyone wants their style to have some staying power so that it lasts longer than a day. Consequently, the blow-dry with a round brush and rollers is what I give them.

A note on terminology: You may have heard the term *blowout* used in your salon or read it in a magazine. Blowout just means to blow-dry. To avoid confusion, I'm going to use only *blow-dry*.

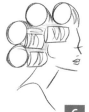

how to 01

BLOW-DRY WITH FINGERS FOR A NATURAL LOOK

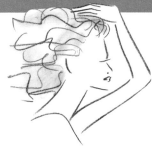

If you want a loose, tousled, "nondone" do that puts very little stress on your hair, this is as easy as it gets!

1 Wash your hair with the shampoo of your choice, condition, towel-dry, and comb.

2 Put 1 or 2 pea-size drops of shine product on your palm; rub your palms together. Starting at the ends and stopping about ½ inch from the roots, blot or squeeze the shine product onto your hair and work it in evenly. With the remaining product traces left on your hands, starting at your forehead, run your hands flat over your hair from front to back.

3 From a distance of 10 inches, spritz a light mist of spray gel all over your hair. Or massage a dime-size or smaller dollop of volumizing gel into your hair, being sure to stop ½ inch from the roots, and follow with a light spritz of volumizing mist.

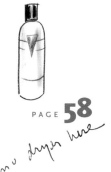

PAGE **58**

no dryer here

4 Flip your head over. To remove moisture and to begin adding volume, lift the roots up from underneath with the fingers of one hand; slowly move your fingers back and forth over your scalp in small movements.

all with head flipped over
LOW SETTING

5 With the blow dryer on a low-heat setting, work the warm air into the roots, drying them quickly as you lift your hair away from your scalp. Do this all over your head just until the roots are damp, not bone dry. If you find the blow dryer is blowing tangles into your hair or blowing your hair around too much, use a diffuser sock over the end of the dryer. You'll be able to remove the moisture from the roots without blowing your hair all around.

6 Switch the blow dryer to a high-heat setting. Flip your head upright.

7 Move the dryer in small circles all over your hair until your hair is completely dry.

8 Arrange your hair with your fingers before further styling and spraying.

PRODUCTS

Shine product

Spray gel or
volumizing gel

Volumizing mist

TOOLS

1600-watt (or higher) blow dryer

Diffuser sock (optional)

BLOW-DRY WITH A DIFFUSER TO ENHANCE CURLY HAIR

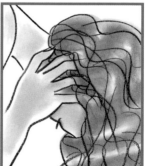

The perfect technique for quick and easy frizz-free curl enhancement.

1   Wash your hair with the shampoo of your choice, condition, towel-dry, and comb.

2   Put 1 or 2 pea-size drops of shine product on your palm; rub your palms together. Starting at the ends and stopping about $\frac{1}{2}$ inch from the roots, blot or squeeze the shine product onto your hair and work it in evenly. With the remaining product traces left on your hands, starting at your forehead, run your hands flat over your hair from front to back.

3   From a distance of 10 inches, spritz a light mist of spray gel all over your hair. Or massage a dime-size or smaller dollop of volumizing gel into your hair, being sure to stop $\frac{1}{2}$ inch from the roots and follow it with a light spritz of volumizing mist. Squeeze curls into your hair by scrunching from ends to roots.

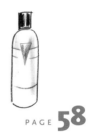

PAGE **58**

4   Flip your head over. To remove moisture and to begin adding volume, lift the roots up from underneath with the fingers of one hand; slowly move your fingers back and forth over your scalp in small movements. Try not to toss your hair around too much, or you'll pull out the curl or cause the curls to frizz.

5   Put the diffuser sock on the blow dryer and switch the dryer onto a low-heat setting. Work the warm air into the roots, drying them quickly as you lift your hair away from your scalp. Do this all over your head just until the roots are damp, not bone dry.

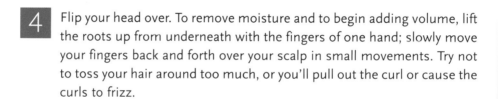

4

6   Switch the blow dryer to a high-heat setting (with diffuser sock still on). Flip your head upright.

7   Working on one section at a time, squeeze curls into your hair by scrunching from ends to roots, following with heat from the blow dryer with a diffuser attachment.

PRODUCTS

Shine product

Spray gel or volumizing gel

Volumizing mist

TOOLS

1600-watt (or higher) blow dryer

Diffuser sock

8   Then, without touching your hair, move the dryer in small circles all over your head until your hair is completely dry.

9   Once your hair is dry, arrange it with your fingers but do not comb or brush it (which will cause your hair to frizz and take the curl out) before further styling and spraying.

ready to roll

ENDS ONTO A ROUND BRUSH

Getting your hair smoothly onto a round brush is half the battle when it comes to mastering blow-dry techniques. If you're already an expert and can roll your hair up from the ends without creating any dreaded fishhooks (caused by not rolling the hair evenly), you can skip these instructions and just get to it. Otherwise, here's an easy way to secure the ends onto the brush. You'll be doing this to blow-dry each section, so it's a good maneuver to know. Hold the round brush in one hand and use the other hand to work with the hair.

1   **Bend** the section (about halfway down its length) over the round brush.

2   **Slide** the brush down the section until you're nearly at the ends.

3   Use your fingers to **tuck** the ends around the brush.

4   **Roll** the brush enough to catch and hold the ends.

5   **Hang** onto the brush with one hand, pick up the blow dryer with the other, and get ready to roll with the heat.

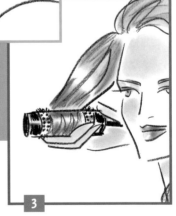

volumizing tip

SPRAY THE HAIR With a single spritz of spray gel at each section after you secure it with the round brush but before you blow-dry it; hold the spray 2 to 3 inches from the hair.

ENDS ONTO A ROLLER

Inserting rollers into your hair smoothly is important for both dry and wet sets. If you're already a pro at rolling from the ends, great. If not, you're in luck because it's really pretty easy. To put in a stick-on roller properly, you secure the ends using a technique similar to that used with a round brush. Be sure not to roll the rollers too tightly, though—they'll get stuck.

1 **Bend** the section (about halfway down its length) over the roller.

2 **Slide** the roller down the section until you're nearly at the ends.

3 Use your fingers to **tuck** the ends around the roller.

4 **Roll** up your hair the rest of the way and clip before moving on to the next section.

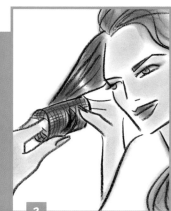

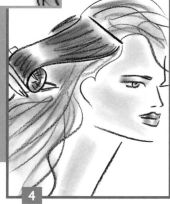

roller tips

LENGTH AND STYLE DETERMINE SIZE The size of the roller you use depends on how long your hair is, how tight you want the curl, and how long you want it to last. The smaller the roller, the tighter the curl and the longer the lasting power. Also, the smaller the roller, the longer the drying time on a wet set.

FIT THE BASE TO THE ROLLER The base is the portion of hair about to be rolled. The width of the base must be the same, or slightly narrower, than that of the roller. If the base is wider than the roller, the hair will spill over the roller ends, and your hairstyle will have random limp pieces.

MINI-SECTIONS MEAN A TIGHTER CURL Depending on the tightness of the curl you want and the sizes of the rollers you choose, you may have to further divide each of "The Big Six" sections into smaller mini-sections. How many mini-sections you use is up to you. When you unclip a section to work on it, use the tail of the rat-tail comb to make the partings for the mini-sections.

how to

BLOW-DRY SMOOTH AND STRAIGHT

This will give you a smooth, flat, glossy shine without volume.

1   Wash your hair with the shampoo of your choice, condition, towel-dry, and comb.

2   Put 1 or 2 pea-size drops of shine product on your palm; rub your palms together. Starting at the ends and stopping about $1/2$ inch from the roots, blot or squeeze the shine product onto your hair and work it in evenly. With the remaining product traces left on your hands, starting at your forehead, run your hands flat over your hair from front to back.

3   Massage a dime-size dollop of straightening pomade into your hair, being sure to stop $1/2$ inch from the roots.

4   Section your hair and clip in place (see pages 72–73). Attach the air-compressor nozzle to your blow dryer and switch onto a high-heat setting.

PAGE **58**

5   If necessary for Section 1 (bangs/front), correct any frizz or cowlick problems with the blow dryer (see page 96). Proceed while Section 1 is still warm.

PAGE **74**

6   On Section 1 (bangs/front), hold the hair with your fingers and pull it down straight. Heat it with the blow dryer, paying special attention to the roots. While the hair is still warm, hold it again with your fingers, pull it down taut, and slowly count to five to let it cool down.

7   Pull down the hair in Section 2 (top/crown) with the fingers of one hand and hold taut. Press the round brush into the roots and pull to create tension. Keep the hair pressed flat against your head with your brush (you can release your fingers) at all times without lifting it up.

8   Follow the brush with the blow dryer and, keeping the nozzle flat against the hair, slide the brush down the section until you reach the ends.

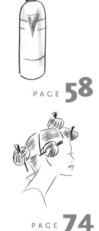

PRODUCTS

Shine product

Straightening pomade

TOOLS

1600-watt (or higher) blow dryer with air-compressor nozzle

Medium-size round brush with perforated metal cylinder

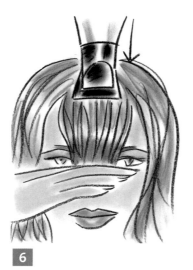

6

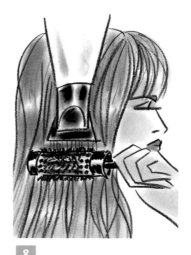

8

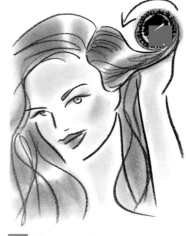

11 if you want the
ends to flip up

9 Repeat the press-pull-slide routine as many times as necessary until the section is dry (3 to 6 times should do it).

10 Repeat Steps 7–9 on Sections 3–6. To create a little height, you may want to insert a large stick-on roller in Section 2 while you dry the back and side sections.

11 Once a section is dry, you can flip the ends by rolling them up (see illustration, top right) slightly in the round brush and blowing with warm air (do not overdirect). Or you can roll them under (see illustration, right) with the round brush and blow with heat (do not overdirect). Or just leave the ends alone.

12 Finish by pressing the roots of Section 1 (bangs/front) flat to your forehead with your hand or fingers and applying a final blast of heat.

13 Add a pea-size amount of straightening pomade for a glossy sheen and to eliminate any frizz.

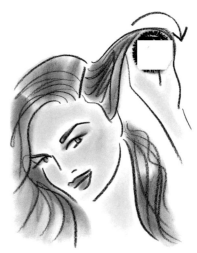

11 if you want the
ends to flip under

how to

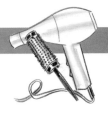

(handwritten margin note) Stop gel ½" from roots

BLOW-DRY WITH A ROUND BRUSH FOR VOLUME

1   Wash your hair with the shampoo of your choice, condition, towel-dry, and comb.

2   Put 1 or 2 pea-size drops of shine product on your palm; rub your palms together. Starting at the ends and stopping about ½ inch from the roots, blot or squeeze the shine product onto your hair and work it in evenly. With the remaining product traces left on your hands, starting at your forehead, run your hands flat over your hair from front to back.

3   From a distance of 10 inches, spritz a light mist of spray gel all over your hair. Or massage a dime-size dollop of volumizing gel into your hair, being sure to stop ½ inch from the roots and follow with a light spritz of volumizing mist.

PAGE **58**

IF YOUR HAIR IS CURLY OR KINKY, apply a small drop of straightening pomade.

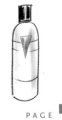

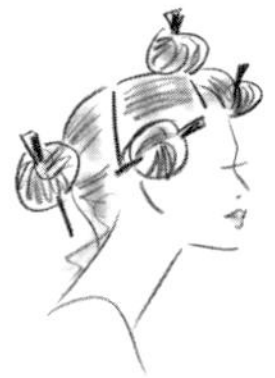

(handwritten margin note) me! →

4   IF YOUR HAIR IS STRAIGHT OR WAVY, flip your head over. To remove moisture and begin adding volume, lift the roots up from underneath with the fingers of one hand; slowly move your fingers back and forth over the scalp in small movements. With the blow dryer on a low-heat setting, work the warm air into the roots, drying them quickly as you lift the hair away from the scalp. Do this all over your head just until the roots are damp, not bone dry. If you find the blow dryer is blowing tangles into your hair, use the diffuser sock over the end of the dryer. You'll be able to remove the moisture from the roots without blowing your hair all around.

PAGE **74**

IF YOUR HAIR IS CURLY OR KINKY, section your hair. Working section by section, with the blow dryer on a low-heat setting and a round brush, work the warm air into the roots, drying them quickly as you lift the hair away from the scalp.

5   Section your hair and clip in place.

PRODUCTS

Shine product

Spray gel or volumizing gel

Straightening pomade (for curly or kinky hair)

Volumizing mist

TOOLS

Wide-tooth comb for sectioning

Clips

1600-watt (or higher) blow dryer

Diffuser sock (optional)

Medium-size round brush with perforated metal cylinder

Wooden styling brush

6   If necessary for Section 1 (bangs/front), correct any frizz and cowlick problems with the blow dryer and fingers (see page 96) and clip in place.

7   Roll the ends of Section 2 (top/crown) onto the round brush. To overdirect the roots, pull the hair in the direction opposite to that in which you want it to lie.

8   With your other hand, switch the blow dryer to high heat. Hold the dryer under the taut hair and blow warm air onto the hair from a distance of 2 to 3 inches.

9   Continuing to overdirect the section, roll and unroll the hair on the round brush a few times. As you do this, warm it with the dryer held 2 to 3 inches underneath for a few seconds, then switch and apply the heat from the top. Alternate back and forth a few times.

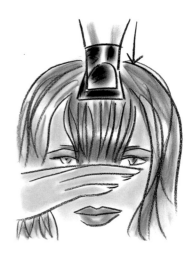

6

10 Repeat the wrap-warm-roll-unroll-release routine as many times as necessary (3 to 6 times should do it) until the section is dry. Be sure to overdirect the hair. Unroll and release the hair from the round brush.

11 Repeat Steps 7–10 on Sections 3–6.

12 Once all the sections are dry, let the hair cool about 10 minutes before further styling. It's the cooling that locks in the body, volume, and style, so don't rush it.

13 Flip your head over and massage the pads of your fingers back and forth all over your scalp to separate the hair. With your head still upside down, very lightly spritz your hair with a fine mist of hairspray, volumizing hairspray, or shaping hairspray; hold the spray 10 to 12 inches from your hair.

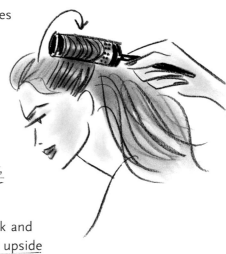

7 overdirect roots, Section 3

14 Flip your head upright. Finish arranging your style with a wooden styling brush.

no more heat
no more heat

how to

POSITION ROLLERS FOR VOLUME: METHOD 1

Use this method for all the hairstyles on pages 106–59 except where you want to set your hair away from your face, as in Half-Up with Wisps (pages 116–17) and Side Sweep (pages 132–33). Read Ready to roll ends onto a roller (page 81) and the drying directions for your chosen style. To begin, brush or comb the hair in each section so you are holding it taut and approximately perpendicular to your scalp.

SECTION 1: BANGS/FRONT Roll your hair back, away from your face. If you have bangs, roll them forward.

SECTION 2: TOP/CROWN Roll your hair back, toward the nape of your neck.

SECTIONS 3 AND 4: LEFT AND RIGHT SIDES Roll your hair down, holding the roller parallel to the floor. If you have short hair, you are finished. If you have medium or long hair, continue rolling the rest of your hair.

SECTIONS 5 AND 6: BACK LEFT AND BACK RIGHT Further divide each of these sections horizontally and vertically so you will be able to use two rows of two rollers for each section. Roll your hair down, holding each roller parallel to the floor.

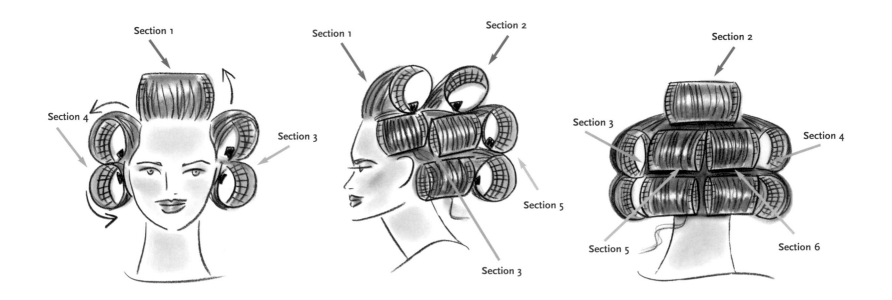

POSITION ROLLERS FOR HAIR SET AWAY FROM THE FACE: METHOD 2

Use this method of inserting rollers for styles where you want to set your hair away from your face like Half-Up with Wisps (pages 116–17) and Side Sweep (pages 132–33). Read Ready to roll ends onto a roller (page 81) and the drying directions for your chosen style. To begin, brush or comb the hair in each section so you are holding it taut and positioned as explained below.

SECTION 1: BANGS/FRONT Hold your hair approximately perpendicular to your scalp. Roll your hair back, away from your face. If you have bangs, roll them forward.

SECTION 2: TOP/CROWN Hold your hair approximately perpendicular to your scalp. Roll your hair back, toward the nape of your neck.

SECTIONS 3 AND 4: LEFT AND RIGHT SIDES Hold your hair approximately perpendicular to your scalp and parallel to the hairline at your temple. Roll your hair back, away from your face.

SECTIONS 5 AND 6: BACK LEFT AND BACK RIGHT Further divide each of these sections vertically so you will be able to use two rollers for each section. Hold your hair taut and angled down. Roll your hair down, holding each roller parallel to the floor; secure each roller at your hairline.

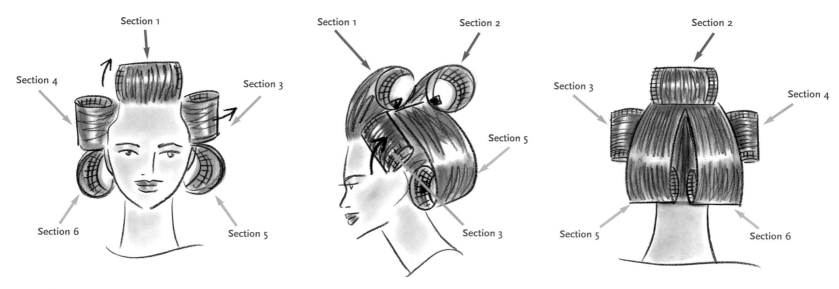

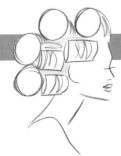

how to

WET-SET FOR VOLUME AND EXTRA HOLD

A wet set is a roller set done on wet hair rather than blow-dried hair. It is still popular for women who desire a tight curl and a super-strong hold and who want to do their hair only once a week. Wet setting is also an excellent way to tame the frizz out of kinky hair.

1. Wash your hair with the shampoo of your choice, condition, towel-dry, and comb.

2. Put 1 to 3 pea-size drops of shine product on your palm; rub your palms together. Starting at the ends and stopping about $\frac{1}{2}$ inch from the roots, blot or squeeze the shine product onto your hair and work it in evenly. With the remaining product traces left on your hands, starting at your forehead, run your hands flat over your hair from front to back.

PAGE **58**

3. Apply gel evenly throughout your hair.

4. Section your hair and clip in place.

PAGE **74**

5. Separate a base for the first roller in Section 1. For extra hold, spray the section with one or two spritzes of setting gel, holding the spray 1 inch from the roots. To overdirect the roots, pull the hair in the direction opposite to that in which you want it to lie. Roll up the base onto the roller and clip. Repeat on the remainder of Section 1.

6. Repeat Step 5 on Sections 2–6.

7. When all your hair is in rollers, mist it with a fine spray of spray gel.

8. There are two options for drying a wet set:

   HOOD DRYER Sit under a hood dryer set at the highest heat setting you can stand. If it is uncomfortable, lower the temperature. Check after 20 to 30 minutes to see if your hair is dry. Longer hair may take more time.

PRODUCTS

Shine product

Setting gel

Spray gel

Hairspray, volumizing hairspray, or shaping hairspray

TOOLS

Wide-tooth comb

Rat-tail comb for mini-sections and back-combing

Clips

Stick-on rollers

Hooded dryer (optional)

Wooden styling brush

NO DRYER This may take some time, but if you have the time, air-drying gives your hair a healthy break from the heat.

9 Allow your hair to cool for 10 minutes before removing the rollers. This helps to set the style and makes it last longer.

10 To remove rollers without tearing your hair, hold the root area of the base with one hand while gently unrolling the roller out with the other.

11 Use a wooden styling brush for styling, or a rat-tail comb for adding extra height and volume. Spritz your hair with a fine mist of hairspray, volumizing hairspray, or shaping hairspray, holding the spray 10 inches from your hair.

wet set tips

KEEP THE SPRAY BOTTLE HANDY If you find that a section is drying out before you get it onto a roller, spritz it with a little water.

SMOOTH RIDGES LATER WITH A DRYER Don't worry if you get some ridges from your wet set. These can easily be corrected with the blow dryer later (see page 97).

ZIGZAG SECTIONING PREVENTS RIDGES This one's for advanced wet setters only (and I know you're out there). Instead of creating the sections with straight parts, use the tail of the rat-tail comb to create zigzag sections.

how to

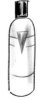

BLOW-DRY WITH A ROUND BRUSH AND ROLLERS

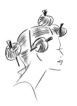

By far and away, this is the most popular styling technique we use in my salon because it's the best for delivering long-lasting volume for all hair types, creating a finished style that is a pleasure to touch, and achieving that beautiful salon look.

1   Wash your hair with the shampoo of your choice, condition, towel-dry, and comb.

2   Put 1 to 3 pea-size drops of shine product on your palm; rub your palms together. Starting at the ends and stopping about $1/2$ inch from the roots, blot or squeeze the shine product onto your hair and work it in evenly. With the remaining product traces left on your hands, starting at your forehead, run your hands flat over your hair from front to back.

PAGE **58**

3   From a distance of 10 inches, spritz a light mist of spray gel all over your hair. Or massage a dime-size dollop of volumizing gel or a golf-ball size dollop of mousse into your hair, being sure to stop $1/2$ inch from the roots, and follow with a light spritz of volumizing mist.

PAGE **74**

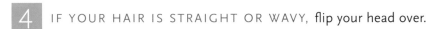

4   IF YOUR HAIR IS STRAIGHT OR WAVY, flip your head over.

IF YOUR HAIR IS CURLY OR KINKY, keep your head upright—otherwise, you risk turning your hair into a frizz bomb.

To remove moisture and begin adding volume, lift the roots up from underneath with the fingers of one hand; slowly move your fingers back and forth over the scalp in small movements.

5   With the blow dryer on a low-heat setting, work the warm air into the roots, drying them quickly as you lift the hair away from the scalp. Do this all over your head just until the roots are damp, not bone dry.

IF YOU HAVE STRAIGHT OR WAVY HAIR and you find the blow dryer is blowing tangles into your hair, use the diffuser sock over the end

PRODUCTS

Shine product

Spray gel, mousse, or volumizing gel

Volumizing mist

Hairspray, volumizing hairspray, or shaping hairspray

TOOLS

Wide-tooth comb for sectioning

Clips

1600-watt (or higher) blow dryer

Diffuser sock (optional)

Medium-size round brush with perforated metal cylinder

Stick-on rollers

Hooded dryer (optional)

Wooden styling brush

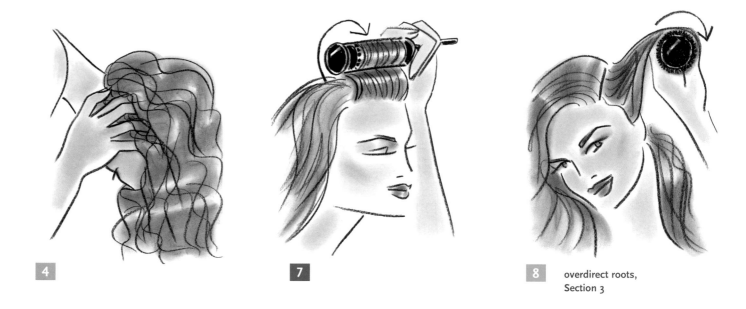

4

7

8 overdirect roots,
Section 3

of the dryer. You'll be able to remove the moisture from the roots without blowing your hair all around.

6 Section your hair and clip in place.

7 If necessary for Section 1 (bangs/front), correct any frizz and cowlick problems with the blow dryer and brush (see page 96) and clip or put in a stick-on roller.

8 Roll the ends of Section 2 (top/crown) onto the round brush. To overdirect the roots, pull the hair in the direction opposite to that in which you want it to lie.

9 With your other hand, switch the blow dryer to high heat. Hold the dryer under the hair and blow warm air onto the hair from a distance of 2 to 3 inches.

10 Continuing to overdirect the section, roll and unroll the hair on the round brush a few times. As you do this, warm it with the dryer held 2 to 3 inches underneath for a few seconds, then switch and apply the heat from the top. Alternate back and forth a few times.

11 Repeat the wrap-warm-roll-unroll-release routine as many times as necessary (3 to 6 times should do it) until the section is dry. Be sure to overdirect the hair. Unroll and release the hair from the round brush.

12 Put the dryer down. While your hair is still warm, and being sure to overdirect the roots, roll in a stick-on roller, secure the ends, roll up, and clip. Doing this while your hair is warm will ensure that the style is set.

13 Repeat Steps 8–13 on Sections 3–6.

14 Once the rollers are positioned and clipped in every section, spritz a light mist of hairspray or spray gel over them all; hold the spray 10 to 12 inches from your head.

15 For extra hold, blow-dry hair in rollers with a diffuser sock or hooded dryer.

16 Leave the rollers in for 10 to 15 minutes before removing them and completing the styling.

17 To remove rollers without tearing your hair, hold the root area of the base with one hand while gently unrolling the roller out with the other.

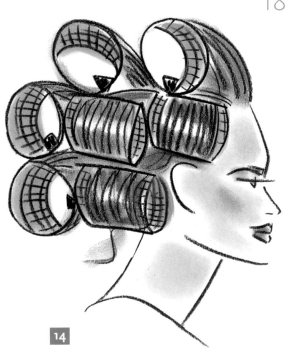

14

18 Flip your head over and massage the pads of your fingers back and forth all over your scalp to separate the hair. With your head still upside down, very lightly spritz your hair with a fine mist of hairspray, volumizing hairspray, or shaping hairspray; hold the spray 10 to 12 inches from your hair.

19 Flip your head upright. Finish arranging your style with a wooden styling brush or comb.

BACK-COMB OR BACK-BRUSH (TEASE) YOUR HAIR

The purpose of teasing—or ratting, matting, or back-combing (all words for the same thing)—is to build a firm base or cushion for extra height or volume. You can do this all over your head or in that one spot (most commonly it's the crown) that needs extra oomph.

Back-brushing accomplishes exactly the same thing that back-combing does, except that the cushioning you create will be soft instead of firm.

Back-combing has the bad reputation of causing split ends, which is what happens if you rip right through the hair. Damage from back-combing can also occur if you do too much of it after using hairspray. To be on the safe side, tease first, spray later.

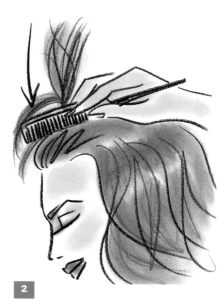

1 Lift a small section of hair (about $3/4$ inch thick) away from the scalp and hold it up firmly with one hand.

2 With your other hand, insert the comb or brush from the back, teeth facing forward, into the lifted hair about $1^{1}/_{2}$ inches above the scalp. Slide the comb or brush down, toward your scalp.

3 Insert the comb or brush further up on the piece (always from the back, teeth facing front) and repeat the sliding down, back-combing motion. I call this shredding.

4 Repeat as many times as necessary, using small, short strokes, until you achieve the cushioning you desire.

5 Gently smooth the hair ends and the top hair over the cushion to hide the back-combing or back-brushing.

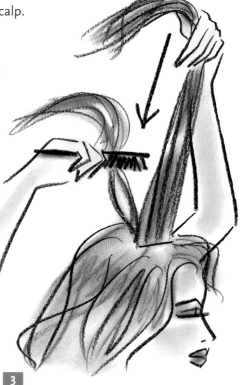

removing back-combing (or brushing) tip

SEPARATE THE HAIR With your fingers, gently separate a few strands of hair at a time. Then, using your fingers like a comb, start at the ends and work toward the roots. Finally, with a wide-tooth comb, start at the ends and gently comb through your hair.

getting it

BIG AND BIGGER

In my salon I like to make hair a lot more voluminous than normal because within an hour it always deflates to the height it should be. If you're going out later, you want your hairstyle to last.

Getting hair bigger is pretty easy. It's just a matter of overdirecting more on the round brush and rollers in the beginning, back-combing more when styling (see previous page), and using more hairspray or spray gel (but always being careful not to use too much). Everything else, from styling to finishing, is exactly the same.

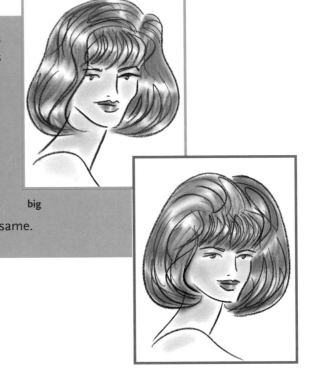

big

bigger

volumizing tips

MAKE IT BIGGER THAN YOU WANT IT No matter how big your hair looks when you first style it, it will settle after a few hours. Furthermore, if you want the body and style to last more than a day, you have to pump up the volume in the beginning. To be on the safe side, overcompensate and create a bit more volume and lift than you ultimately want.

FLIP IT After your hair is completely dry, flip your head over and gently pull your hair away from the scalp with your fingers in a lift and rake motion, section by section, but without pulling your fingers all the way through to the ends.

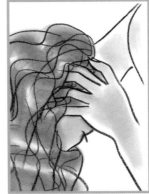

flip head over, rake hair

Finishing techniques

Finishing is a hairdresser's term for a making sure a hairstyle is perfectly in balance from every direction. Finishing means checking for and correcting any flyaways, frizzies, clumps, or holes and being sure that any back-combing is hidden within the structure of the style rather than sticking out and looking ratty. Finishing is what separates the amateurs from the pros.

Intentionally messy looks can be finished too; it's the balance that's the key.

The first key to finishing is to train your eye to look at your hair and really see it accurately from every direction. Your hair may look perfect head on in the mirror, but life, my dear, is three-dimensional. What looks even in front may, in fact, be lopsided or crooked in profile. Invest in a good hand mirror that is large enough to give you a view of your whole head from every angle. As time goes on, you'll find that practice makes your eye sharper.

Here's a list of things you should check to be sure that your style is finished. Look in a hand mirror to see the back and sides of your head in the bathroom mirror.

- The left and right sides match up.

- The ends fall evenly all the way around.

- There are no holes or clumps on the top, back, or sides.

- No back-combing shows from the top, back, or sides.

The good news about finishing is that if something isn't quite the way you want it, you can easily fix it. These techniques should help you get pretty close to a finished salon look.

how to

TAME A DIFFICULT HAIRLINE OR COWLICK

Section 1 (bangs/front) is especially prone to frizz (although frizz can occur any-where) and cowlicks (although you can have them anywhere too). Tension and the air-compressor nozzle on the blow dryer are what it takes to wrangle those stubborn spots into place. When taming, apply styling product before drying. This technique works best for wet hair immediately after washing it if it is frizzy or cowlicky. It can also be used on dry hair between shampoos or as a touch up.

1 Move the troublesome hair from left to right with a round brush (or with your fingers, whichever is easier for you) and pull it taut. With the blow dryer (with or without the air-compressor nozzle) on the highest heat setting, heat the roots for a few seconds; keep a small amount of tension on the hair as you do this.

2 Immediately move the hair in the opposite direction, from right to left, with the round brush (or fingers) and hold it taut that way. Heat the roots for a few seconds.

3 Alternate Steps 1 and 2 until the section is dry.

4 FOR VOLUME AND LIFT After correcting frizz or a cowlick and while your hair is still warm, follow the directions for How to Blow-Dry with Round Brush (see pages 84–85), using more tension in the areas that tend to get frizzy. Or just put in a stick-on roller and allow your hair to cool down for 10 minutes.

FOR FLAT BANGS After correcting frizz or a cowlick, follow the direc-tions for How to Blow-Dry Smooth and Straight (see pages 82–83). Finish by working your fingertips to the base of the roots and rubbing back and forth a couple of times. Comb or brush your bangs down and then hold them down with the flat of your hand. Hit the roots with a final blast of heat. Hold your warm bangs flat for a few seconds as they cool down.

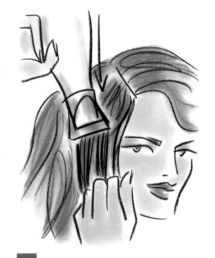

1

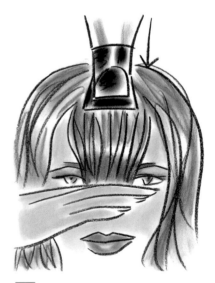

4 for flat bangs

SMOOTH OUT RIDGES ON STRAIGHT HAIR

1 Follow exactly the same procedure as you would to Tame a Difficult Hairline or Cowlick (opposite page).

2 The key is to break the direction of the ridge by moving the hair from left to right as you pull it taut and heat it with the blow dryer at the base of the root.

SMOOTH OUT RIDGES ON CURLY HAIR FROM A WET SET

1 Put the blow dryer on the high-heat setting with the diffuser sock on.

2 Dampen your fingers. Then, using the pads of your fingertips, massage the area gently against the grain of the ridge as you heat it with the blow dryer.

TAME STATIC

1 Put a pea-size drop of shine product on your palm (too much will weigh the hair down) and rub your palms together.

2 Run your fingers through your hair wherever there is static.

Trimming your own bangs

I love the look of bangs because they're very youthful and can add some versatility to a hairstyle. As for length, I like bangs that look natural but aren't too short—the way they were when your mother got hold of them and cut them when you were a kid. This means long or short, whatever you like, but just not *too* short.

It can often seem like your bangs grow out too quickly—certainly faster than you can get to the hairdresser. Your bangs usually need a little snip about the third or fourth week after a haircut. While it is taboo to cut your own hair, if your bangs are making you absolutely crazy, you can carefully trim them yourself using little haircutting scissors (available at beauty supply stores). But be careful and snip off only a little at a time. Your bangs didn't grow *that* much, and you can always go back and take off a little more later. Always work in $1/4$-inch increments.

The one thing I tell people is always to trim your bangs longer than you want them. Whether you trim them wet or dry is up to you. Whichever you choose, remember that the hair is *always* going to jump shorter than when you cut it. This goes for straight hair as well as curly, wavy, and kinky hair.

To trim your bangs, first section off the bangs area and clip the rest of your hair out of the way. Then, choose which look you want below and follow the instructions:

FOR A FLATTERING ROUNDED LOOK Pull your bangs down and together to meet in the middle with one hand. Trim straight across with the other hand.

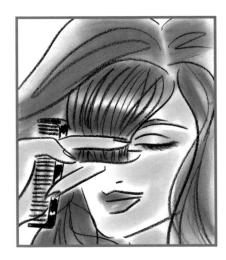 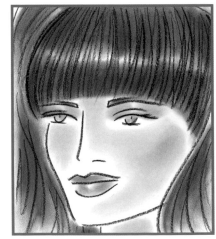

FOR A BLUNT-CUT LOOK Pull your bangs straight down with one hand and snip straight across with the other.

FOR A WISPY LOOK Pull your bangs down and together to meet in the middle with one hand. Trim with the other. Cut up into your bangs to make jagged edges. (You can use this technique on rounded or blunt-cut bangs.)

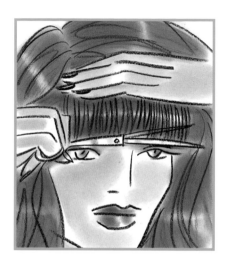 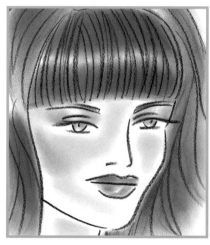 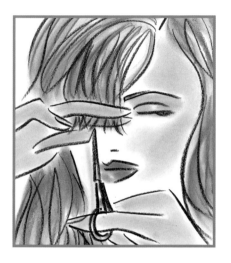

bangs trimming tips

TRIMMING STRAIGHT HAIR I usually suggest trimming dry hair to just below the eyebrows. The bangs will jump to the top of the eyebrows once they're styled. Trim wet hair to the middle of the bridge of the nose so the bangs will dry to eyebrow length.

TRIMMING WAVY OR CURLY HAIR I prefer to trim wavy or curly bangs when wet (frizzy bangs should be left to your hairdresser). I like to trim them to the tip of the nose so the bangs will dry to eyebrow length. If you have a cowlick, trim the side with the cowlick to be slightly longer than the side without.

TRIMMING BANGS WITH A COWLICK I suggest you blow dry bangs first. Let bangs set for a minute or two, and then trim them slightly.

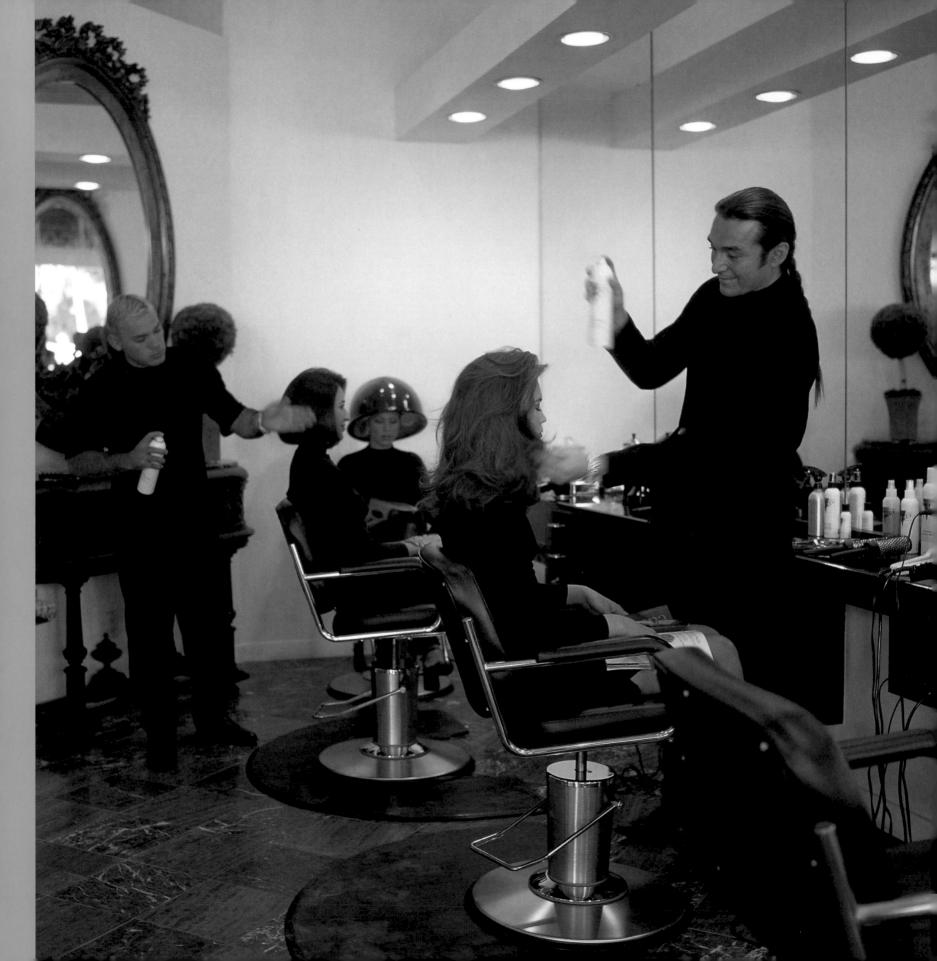

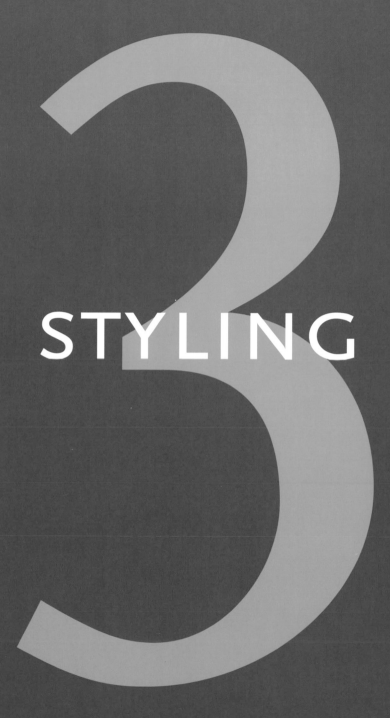

STYLING

3

all about
straight hair

If you have straight hair with a good haircut and you wash and condition it properly, your hair can look great without too much work. Of all the hair types, straight hair (when it's healthy, that is) reflects light the most easily, which is what makes it shine.

If you have straight hair and you like precision blunt cuts and letting your hair air-dry, you're lucky. A more tousled look requires a haircut with layers. When it comes to haircuts, though, straight hair can be very unforgiving; it doesn't have any wave or curl to disguise cutting mistakes or inaccuracies.

Straight hair's major disadvantage is that it usually doesn't hold a curl very well. And if your hair is straight and limp, it doesn't have much natural body. The solution is to use a round brush with a perforated metal cylinder and stick-on rollers—not for curl necessarily, but for body, lift, and volume.

Setting straight hair

To set straight hair with a blow dryer, round brush, and stick-on rollers, you really have to remember to heat up the hair thoroughly while it's on the brush (the brush's metal cylinder will help with this a lot). Then, immediately insert the rollers to help it curl. Otherwise, the curl won't hold. And if your hair is naturally board straight, with absolutely no bend in it at all, leave the rollers in for 20 minutes (as opposed to the usual 10 to 15) to make sure the curl really sets. Wet sets and hood drying give straight hair the strongest, longest-lasting curls of all.

After removing the rollers, if you want your hair to have body without curl, brush it out and style it. If you want the curls to hold, just use your fingers to pull at the hair very lightly as you style, but do not brush or comb it. Whether you

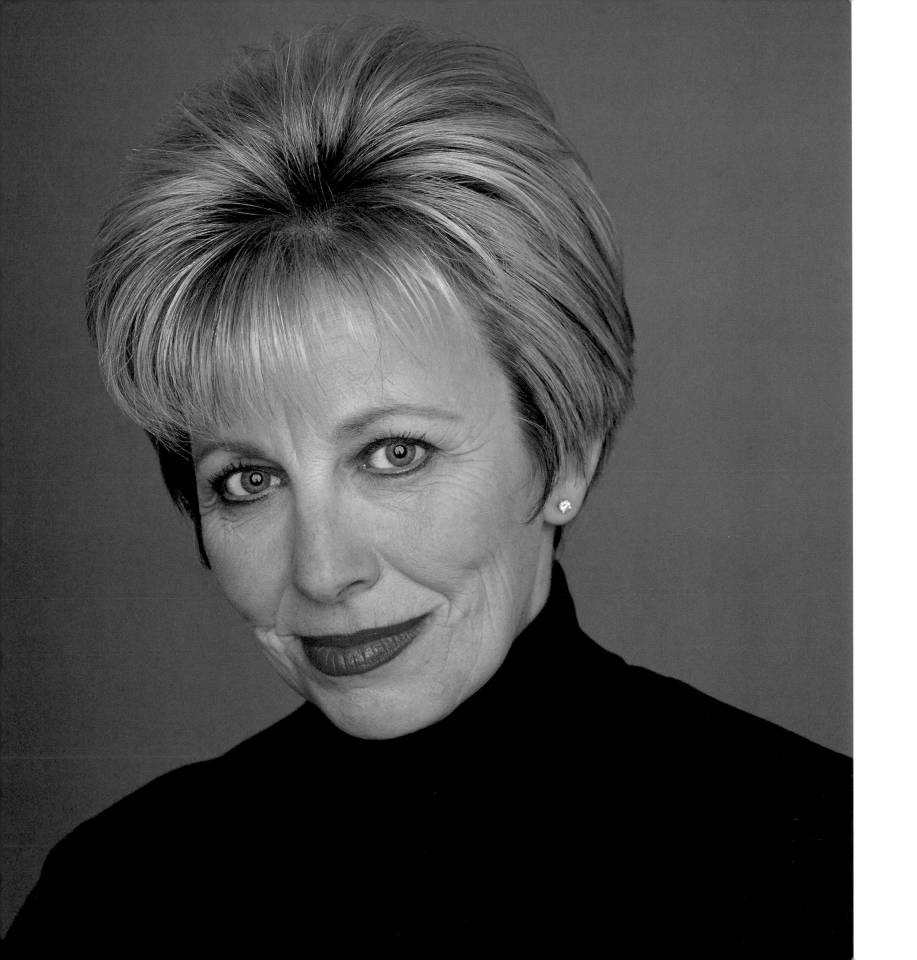

want curls or not, flipping your head over as you style your hair adds body (pulling the roots away from the scalp is what helps creates the volume), as do volumizing products.

Straight thin hair

My clients with straight thin hair (which is frequently fine and limp also) want fullness. Even if they wear it straight and blunt in a bob, they want it to seem thick. Volumizing products will help, as will flipping the head upside down during the initial stages of the blow-dry.

Be sure to shampoo and rinse straight thin hair thoroughly; if this type of hair isn't washed and rinsed thoroughly, you will be able to see the scalp through the hair.

Straight thick hair

Straight thick hair always looks good. Its primary disadvantage is that it can take a long time to dry and it might not hold a curl because it can be stubborn and heavy. Otherwise, it's terrific hair to have. Volumizing products are great for lifting heavy hair away from the scalp.

1 Wash your hair with the shampoo of your choice, condition, towel-dry, and comb.

2 Blow-dry your hair with a round brush and rollers; set on rollers using Method 1 (see page 86), but roll only the crown of your head. Leave the rollers in for 10 to 15 minutes and then remove gently.

3 Brush your hair out. Back-comb for a little extra height.

4 Arrange with your fingers or a wooden styling brush.

5 Finish with a light mist of hairspray.

good for

SHORT TO MEDIUM-LENGTH STRAIGHT HAIR

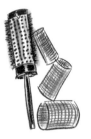

PAGE **58**

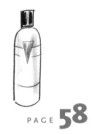

PAGE **90**

PRODUCTS

Hairspray, volumizing hairspray, or shaping hairspray

TOOLS

1600-watt (or higher) blow dryer

Medium-size round brush with perforated metal cylinder

Medium-size (green) stick-on rollers

Wooden styling brush

Fine-tooth or wide-tooth comb

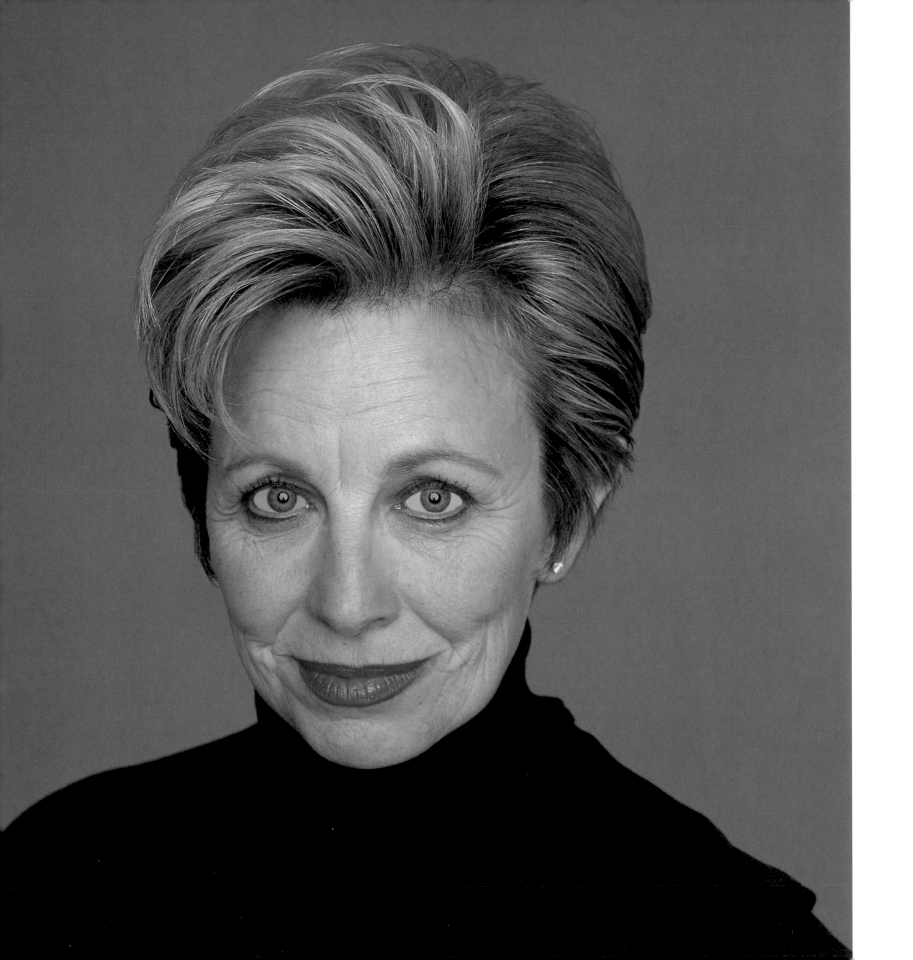

short sweep

1 Wash your hair with the shampoo of your choice, condition, towel-dry, and comb.

2 Blow-dry your hair with a round brush and rollers; set on rollers using Method 2 (see page 87). Leave the rollers in for 10 to 15 minutes and then remove gently.

3 Spray your hair all over with spray gel or hairspray or rub a nickel-size dollop of sculpting gel or volumizing gel onto your palms and then into your hair, running your fingers completely through your hair.

4 Press the hair at the sides of your head closer to your face. You may want to rub another pea-size drop of gel on your hair to get the hold you need.

5 Style and arrange pieces with your fingers, pulling the bang area back and to the side.

6 Use a blow dryer with a diffuser sock to lock in the hair style.

7 Finish with a light mist of hairspray.

good for

SHORT TO
MEDIUM-LENGTH
STRAIGHT HAIR

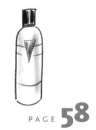

PAGE **58**

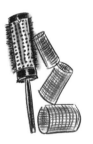

PAGE **90**

PRODUCTS

Spray gel, sculpting gel, or volumizing gel

Hairspray, volumizing hairspray, or shaping hairspray

TOOLS

1600-watt (or higher) blow dryer

Medium-size round brush with perforated metal cylinder

Medium-size (green) and small (red) stick-on rollers

Diffuser sock

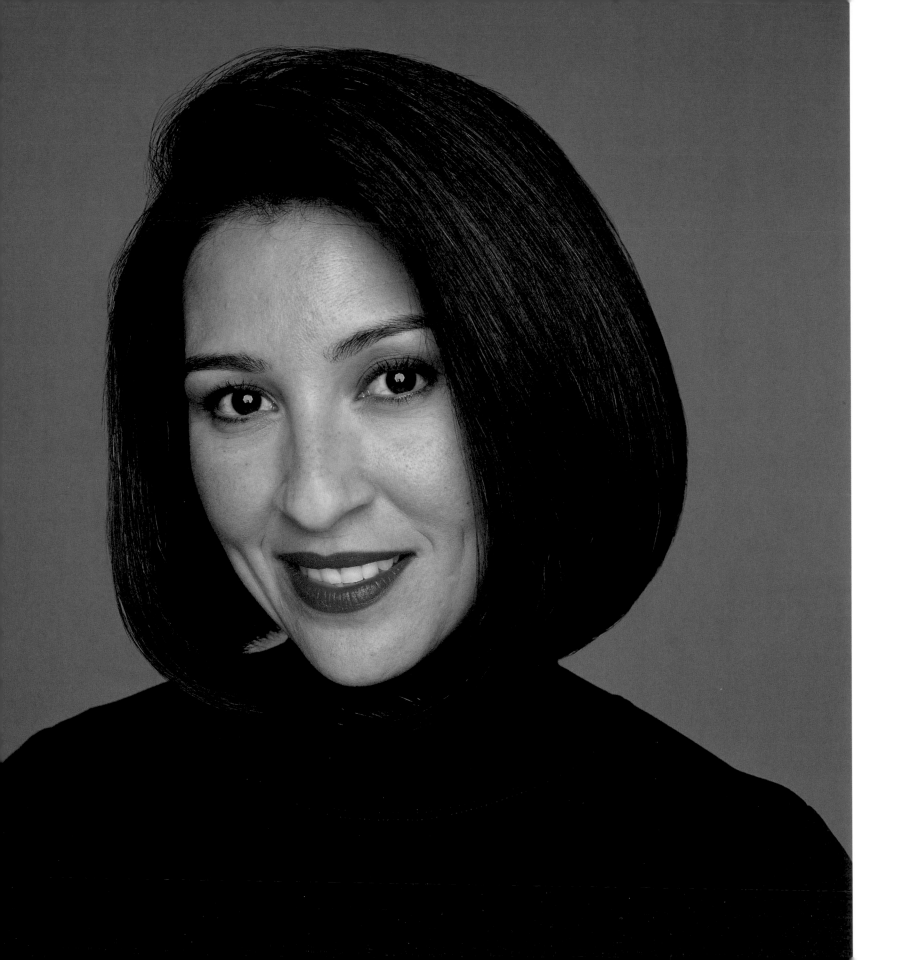

perfect bob

1 Wash your hair with the shampoo of your choice, condition, towel-dry, and comb.

2 Blow-dry your hair with a round brush and rollers; set on rollers using Method 1 (see page 86). Leave the rollers in for 10 to 15 minutes and then remove gently.

3 Brush your hair out.

4 Comb your hair into place, sweeping the top to one side.

5 Finish with a light mist of hairspray.

good for

SHORT TO
MEDIUM-LENGTH
STRAIGHT HAIR

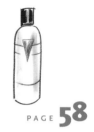

PAGE **58**

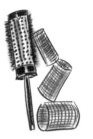

PAGE **90**

see page 86

PRODUCTS

Hairspray, volumizing hairspray, or shaping hairspray

TOOLS

1600-watt (or higher) blow dryer

Medium-size round brush with perforated metal cylinder

Large (blue) stick-on rollers

Wooden styling brush

Fine-tooth or wide-tooth comb

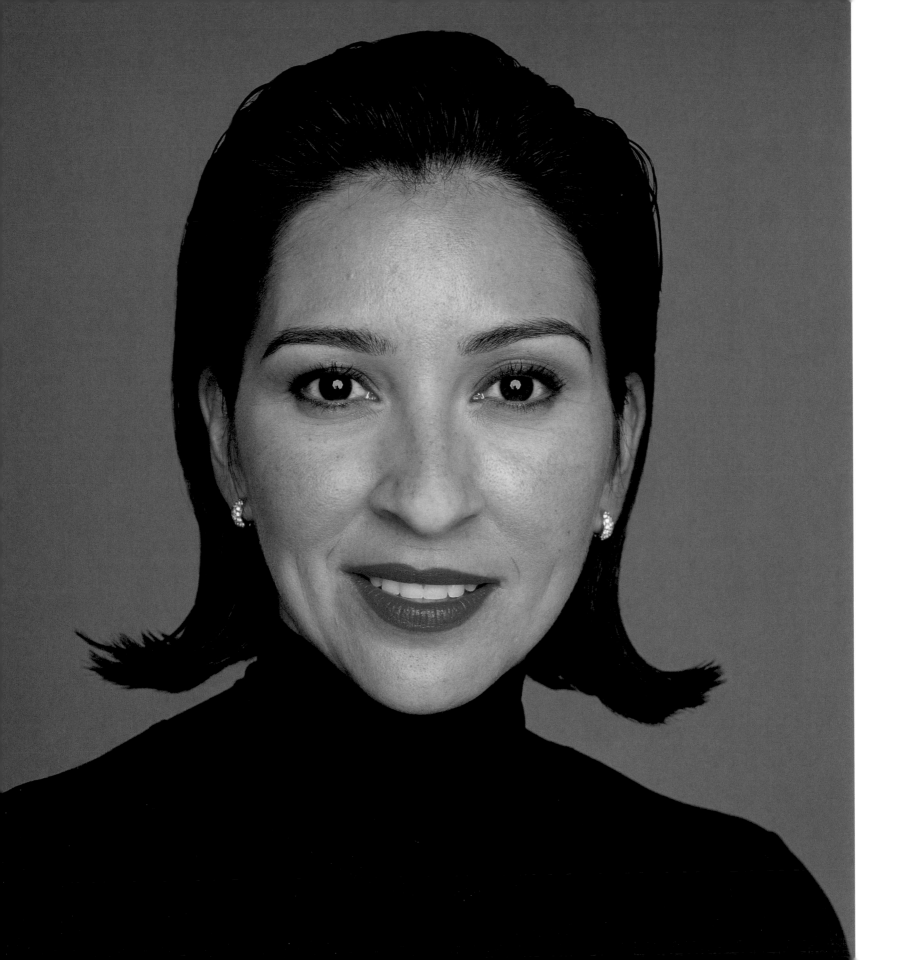

refined flip

1 Wash your hair with the shampoo of your choice, condition, towel-dry, and comb.

2 Rub a quarter-size dollop of sculpting gel or volumizing gel between your palms and work the gel into your hair, or thoroughly spray your hair with spray gel.

3 Slick back your hair and style it with a comb or your fingers. Turn the hair up (sculpt it) with your fingers. If your hair has a natural flip or your hair-cut encourages a flip, you won't need to use much product. Otherwise, you may need to use a little bit more gel. For a more defined flip, roll the ends up in a round brush (not overdirecting) and hit them underneath with a blast of high heat from the blow dryer.

4 Blow-dry your hair using a diffuser sock to dry your hair and lock in style.

5 (optional) Finish with a light mist of hairspray.

good for

SHORT TO MEDIUM-LENGTH STRAIGHT HAIR

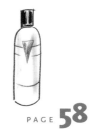

PAGE **58**

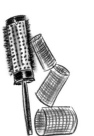

PAGE **90**

PAGE 58

PAGE 90

PRODUCTS

Sculpting gel, volumizing gel, or spray gel

Hairspray, volumizing hairspray, or shaping hairspray (optional)

TOOLS

Fine-tooth or wide-tooth comb (optional)

Medium-size round brush with perforated metal cylinder (optional)

1600-watt (or higher) blow dryer

Diffuser sock

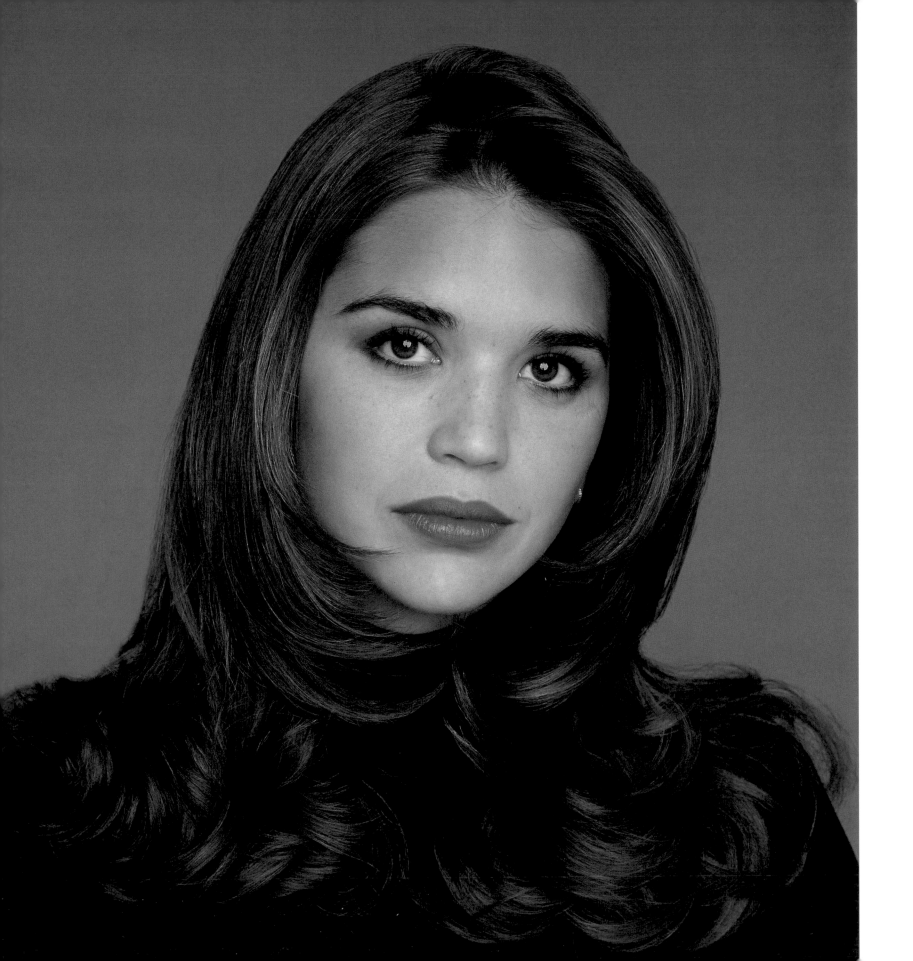

silken waves

1 Wash your hair with the shampoo of your choice, condition, towel-dry, and comb.

2 Blow-dry your hair with a round brush and rollers; set on rollers using Method 1 (see page 86). Leave the rollers in for 10 to 15 minutes and then remove gently.

3 Flip your head over. Work your fingers over your scalp to loosen the curl. Do not brush.

4 With your head still down, lightly mist your hair with hairspray.

5 Flip your head upright.

6 Arrange your hair with your fingers or a comb. (Optional: create a zigzag part.)

7 Finish with a light mist of hairspray.

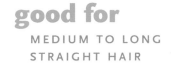

good for
MEDIUM TO LONG STRAIGHT HAIR

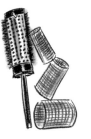

PAGE **58**

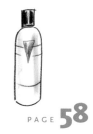

PAGE **90**

PRODUCTS

Hairspray, volumizing hairspray, or shaping hairspray

TOOLS

1600-watt (or higher) blow dryer

Medium-size round brush with perforated metal cylinder

Medium-size (green) stick-on rollers

Fine-tooth or wide-tooth comb (optional)

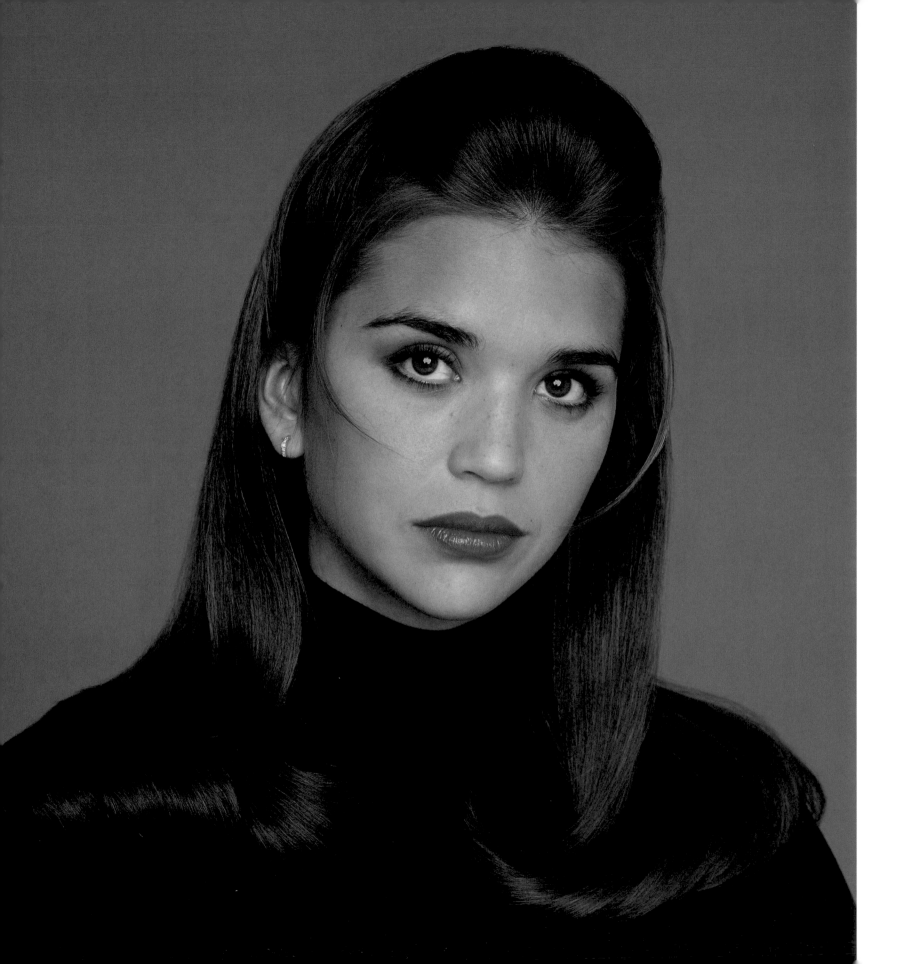

half-up with wisps

1 Wash your hair with the shampoo of your choice, condition, towel-dry, and comb.

2 Blow-dry your hair with a round brush and rollers; set on rollers using Method 2 (see page 87). Leave the rollers in for 10 to 15 minutes and then remove gently.

3 Brush your hair out.

4 (optional) Pull out wisps of hair at the sides.

5 Using the top of your ear as your guide, use a comb to create an upward-slanting horizontal part on each side; gather up the hair above the part in one hand.

6 With that same hand, twist the hair once, then twist it again.

7 Still holding the twisted hair in the same hand, push it forward slightly to get volume into the front. Secure with bobby pins or a barrette.

8 Finish with a light mist of hairspray.

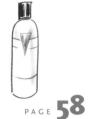

PAGE **58**

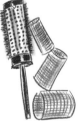

PAGE **90**

PRODUCTS

Hairspray, volumizing hairspray, or shaping hairspray

TOOLS

1600-watt (or higher) blow dryer

Medium-size round brush with perforated metal cylinder

Medium-size (green) stick-on rollers

Wooden styling brush

Fine-tooth or wide-tooth comb

Bobby pins or barrette

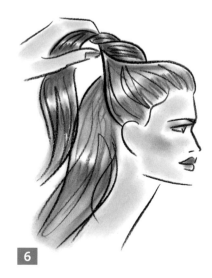

6

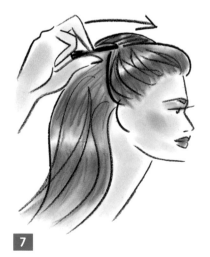

7

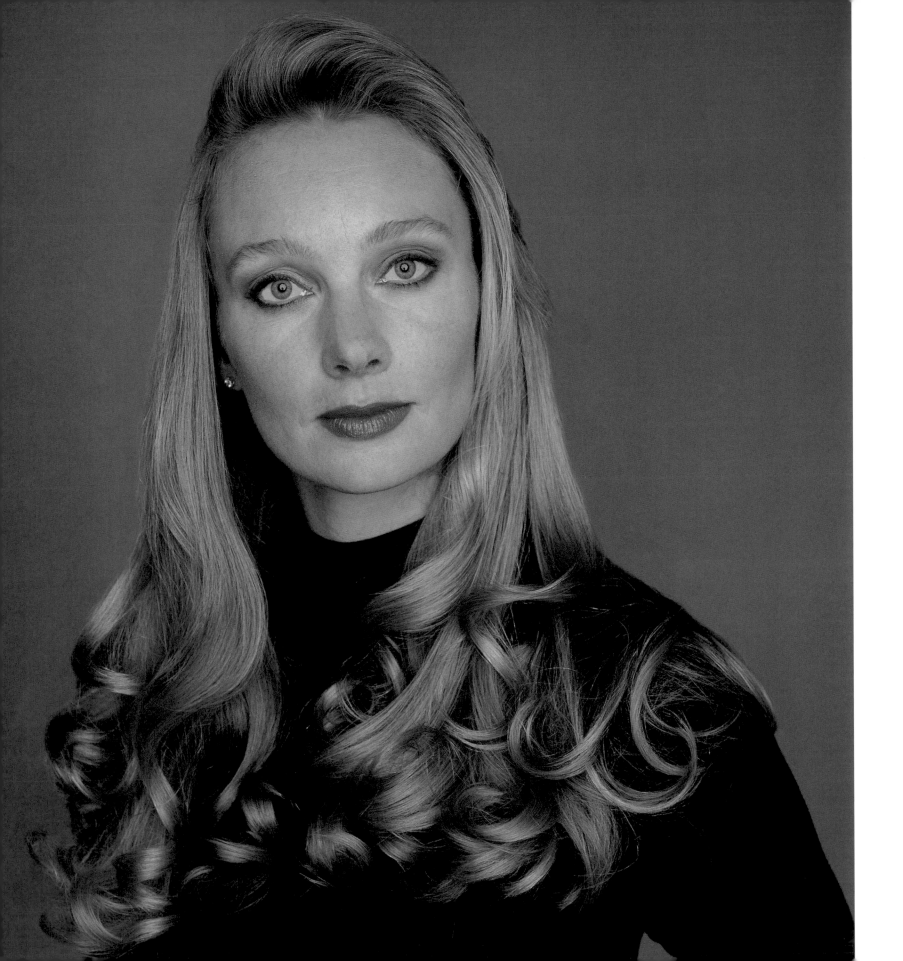

mermaid

good for

MEDIUM TO LONG
STRAIGHT HAIR

1 Wash your hair with the shampoo of your choice, condition, towel-dry, and comb.

2 Blow dry your hair with a round brush and rollers; set on rollers using Method 1 (see page 86). Leave the rollers in for 10 to 15 minutes.

3 Gently remove the rollers, one at a time, lightly spraying each curl with hairspray and then letting it fall. Do not brush.

4 When all the rollers are out and each curl is individually sprayed, divide the coil of each curl by pulling it apart with your fingers to create smaller and more abundant curls.

5 Arrange the ends of your hair with your fingers. Lift your bangs up and slightly back-comb them to the side.

6 Finish with a light mist of hairspray.

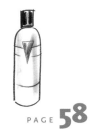

PAGE **58**

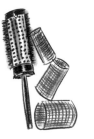

PAGE **90**

PRODUCTS

Hairspray, volumizing hairspray, or shaping hairspray

TOOLS

1600-watt (or higher) blow dryer

Medium-size round brush with perforated metal cylinder

Small (red) stick-on rollers

Fine-tooth or wide-tooth comb

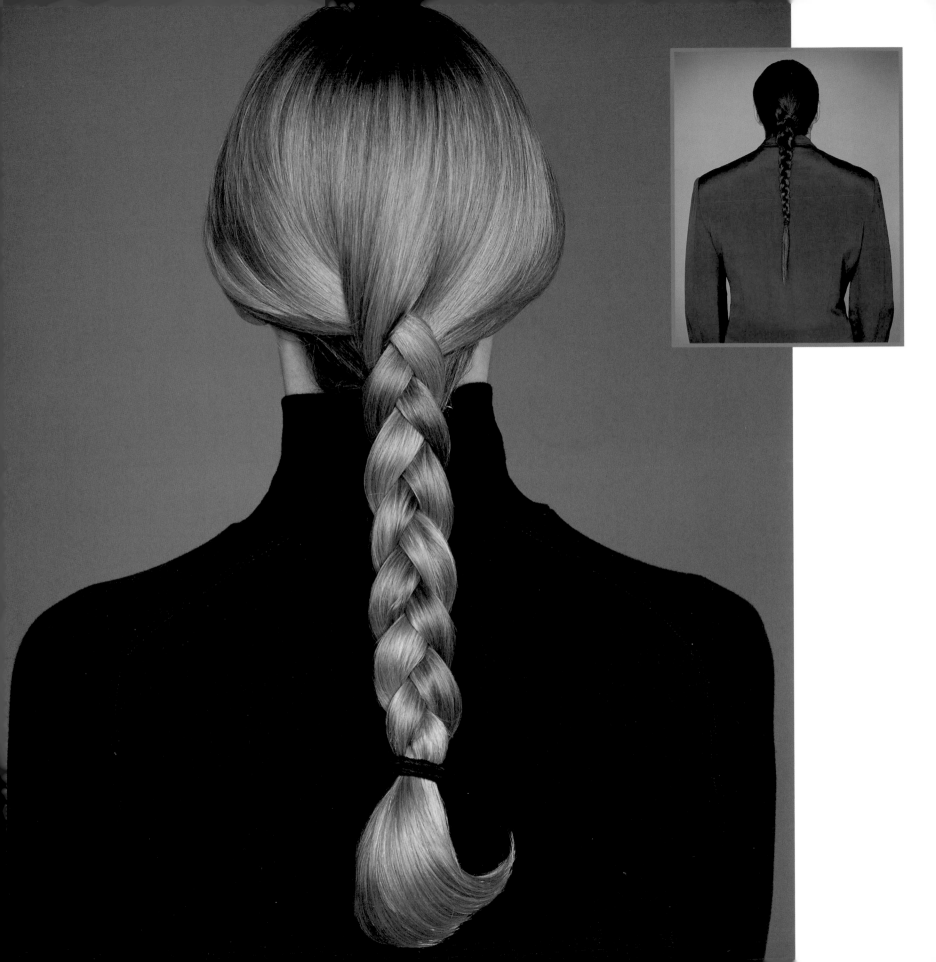

chavez braid

This inside-out braid is how I wear my hair everyday (see inset).

good for

MEDIUM TO LONG
STRAIGHT HAIR

1 Wash your hair with the shampoo of your choice, condition, towel-dry, and comb.

2 Blow-dry your hair with a round brush.

3 Brush your hair out.

4 If you have flyaways, *lightly* mist with spray gel or hairspray here, otherwise you can skip this step. Pay extra attention to make sure the front hairline and top of the head are smooth.

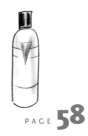

PAGE **58**

5 (optional) Pull out any wisps at the sides you don't want braided.

6 At the nape of the neck, divide your hair into three equal sections.

7 Working with both hands, braid your hair from underneath: Take the section on the right and weave it under the middle section so that it becomes the middle section. Then, take the section on the left and weave it under the middle section so that it becomes the middle section. Continue weaving the right and left sections underneath the middle section until you have braided all your hair.

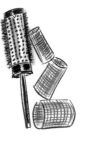

PAGE **90**

8 Secure with a covered elastic band at the end.

9 Finish with a light mist of hairspray.

PRODUCTS

Spray gel (optional)

Hairspray, volumizing hairspray, or shaping hairspray

TOOLS

1600-watt (or higher) blow dryer

Medium-size round brush with perforated metal cylinder

Wooden styling brush

Covered elastic band

all about
wavy hair

Wavy hair is the most versatile of all the hair types because you can set it in a tight curl or you can blow-dry it straight. Naturally wavy hair gives you a lot more volume than straight hair does, and once it is styled, it holds curl and body for a long time.

Wavy hair tends to assume a pyramid shape (narrow at the crown and flaring out around the ears) if it's cut in a blunt cut. Some people like this shape but most do not because it can look boxy at the jawline. Layered cuts bring out the waves to best advantage.

The downside to wavy hair is that it can frizz at times. Correct product use will go a long way toward preventing or removing frizz from wavy hair. One great frizz-busting trick is to mix shine product and spray gel together (but be careful not to use too much; just the finest film on your hands is what you're after) and work it through the ends evenly.

To add body, volumizing products are key, as is working upside down in the preliminary steps of the blow-dry. (Working upside down separates the roots away from the scalp, which is what creates volume.) Scrunching while blow-drying is an easy way to get tighter curl into wavy hair if you don't want to set it. To maintain curl after setting or scrunching, do not comb or brush your hair, but arrange it with your fingers as you style.

Wavy thin hair

The good news is that because of the bend formation, wavy thin hair looks thicker than it actually is. The not-so-good news is that wavy thin hair tends to get a little frizzy at the ends. Go easy on styling products if you have wavy thin hair. Using too much product will plaster your hair down, allowing others to see your scalp.

Wavy thick hair

This is great hair because it has a beautiful wave to it, looks thick, and has lots of volume on its own. The downside of wavy thick hair is that your scalp can get really oily if you don't use the right products. Plus, if you don't wash and rinse it properly, hair this thick can trap a lot of a product, leading to dull, lifeless hair and a flaky scalp.

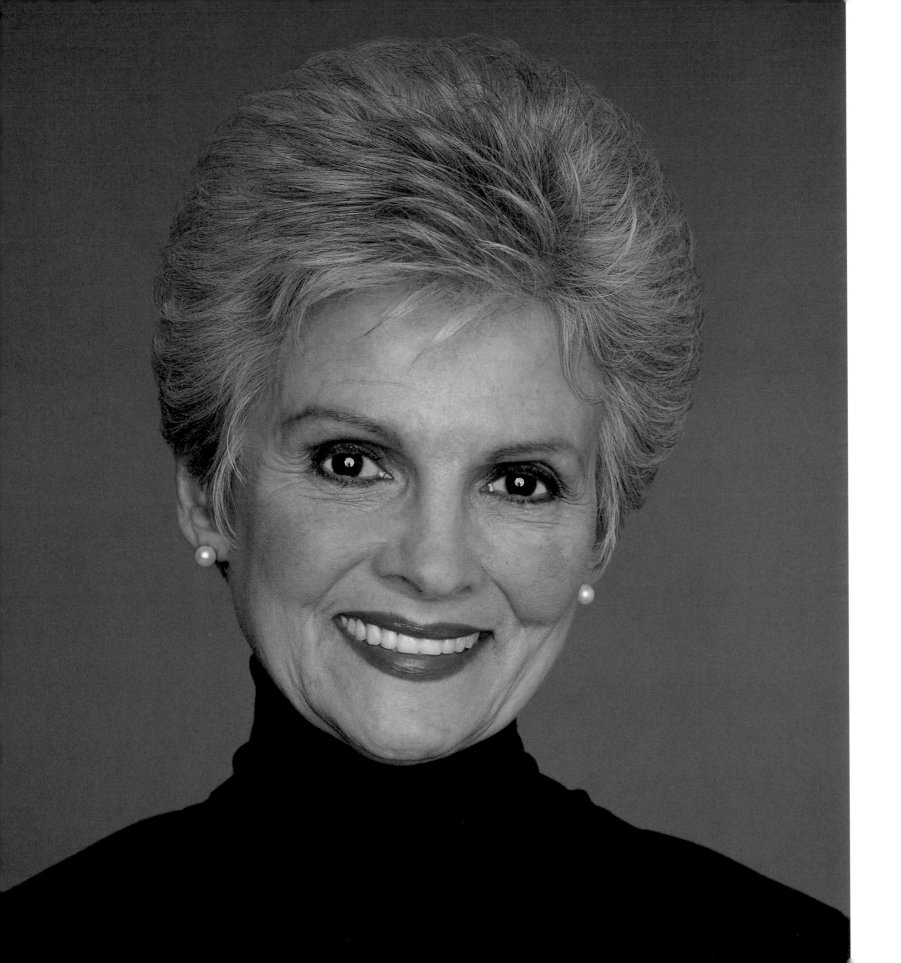

1 Wash your hair with the shampoo of your choice, condition, towel-dry, and comb.

2 Blow-dry your hair with a round brush and rollers; set on rollers using Method 2 (see page 87). Leave the rollers in for 10 to 15 minutes and then remove gently.

3 For extra volume at the crown, back-comb your hair slightly.

4 Brush your hair to the side into place or use your fingers to style it.

5 Finish with a light mist of hairspray.

good for

SHORT TO
MEDIUM-LENGTH
WAVY HAIR

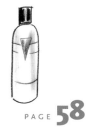

PAGE **58**

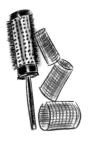

PAGE **90**

PRODUCTS

Hairspray, volumizing
hairspray, or shaping
hairspray

TOOLS

1600-watt (or higher)
blow dryer

Medium-size round brush
with perforated metal cylinder

Small (red) stick-on rollers

Fine-tooth or wide-tooth comb

Wooden styling brush
(optional)

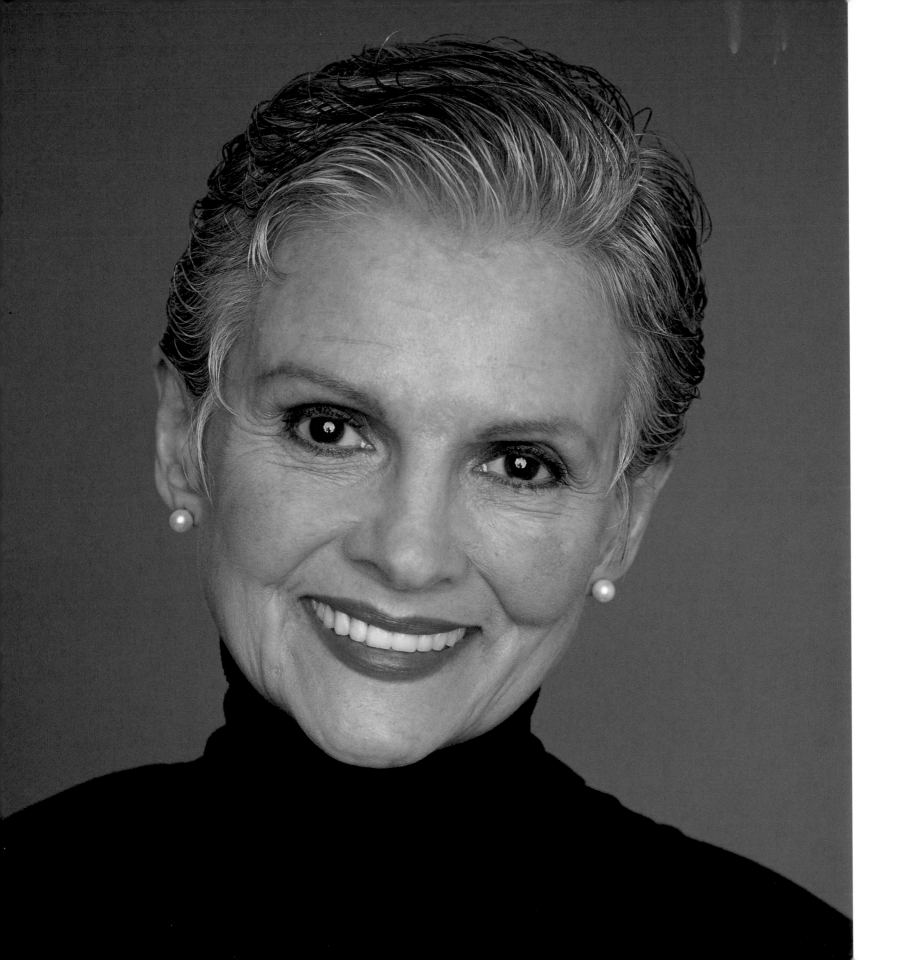

sleek and chic

good for

SHORT TO
MEDIUM-LENGTH
WAVY HAIR

1 Wash your hair with the shampoo of your choice, condition, towel-dry, and comb.

2 Rub a nickel-size dollop of sculpting gel or volumizing gel between your palms and work the gel into your hair, or thoroughly spray your hair with spray gel.

3 Slick back your hair and style it with a comb or your fingers. Create a side part if desired.

4 Use a blow dryer with a diffuser sock to dry your hair and lock in style.

5 (optional) Finish with a light mist of hairspray.

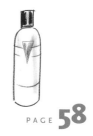

PAGE **58**

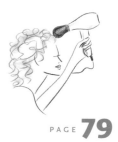

PAGE **79**

Just 1 product

PRODUCTS

Sculpting gel, volumizing gel, or spray gel

Hairspray, volumizing hairspray, or shaping hairspray (optional)

TOOLS

Fine-tooth or wide-tooth comb (optional)

1600-watt (or higher) blow dryer

Diffuser sock

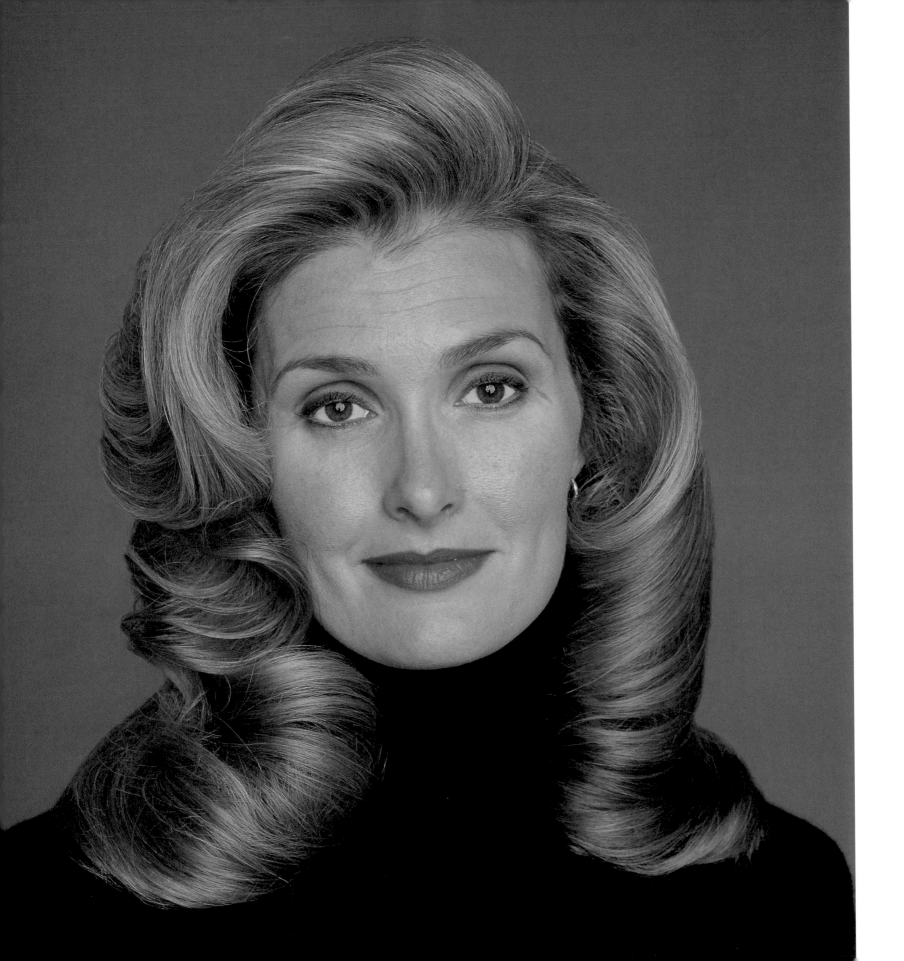

hollywood

1 Wash your hair with the shampoo of your choice, condition, towel-dry, and comb.

2 Set your wet hair on rollers using Method 1 (see page 86) and dry under a hood dryer on high-heat setting for 30 to 45 minutes, depending on the thickness of your hair. When your hair is completely dry, gently remove the rollers.

3 Brush your hair out. Use a comb to create a part if desired.

4 Brush the sides and roll them under, using your fingers to position the curls so they coil the way you want them to.

5 Place one hand flat on top of your head and push your hair slightly back and then forward to get lift in front. While pushing your hair forward, lightly mist the front with hairspray for a firmer hold.

6 Finish with a light mist of hairspray.

good for
MEDIUM TO LONG WAVY HAIR

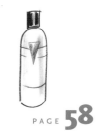

PAGE **58**

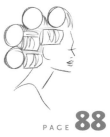

PAGE **88**

PRODUCTS

Hairspray, volumizing hairspray, or shaping hairspray

TOOLS

Medium-size (green) stick-on rollers

Hooded dryer

Wooden styling brush

Fine-tooth or wide-tooth comb (optional)

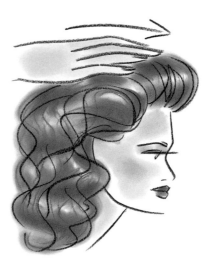

5

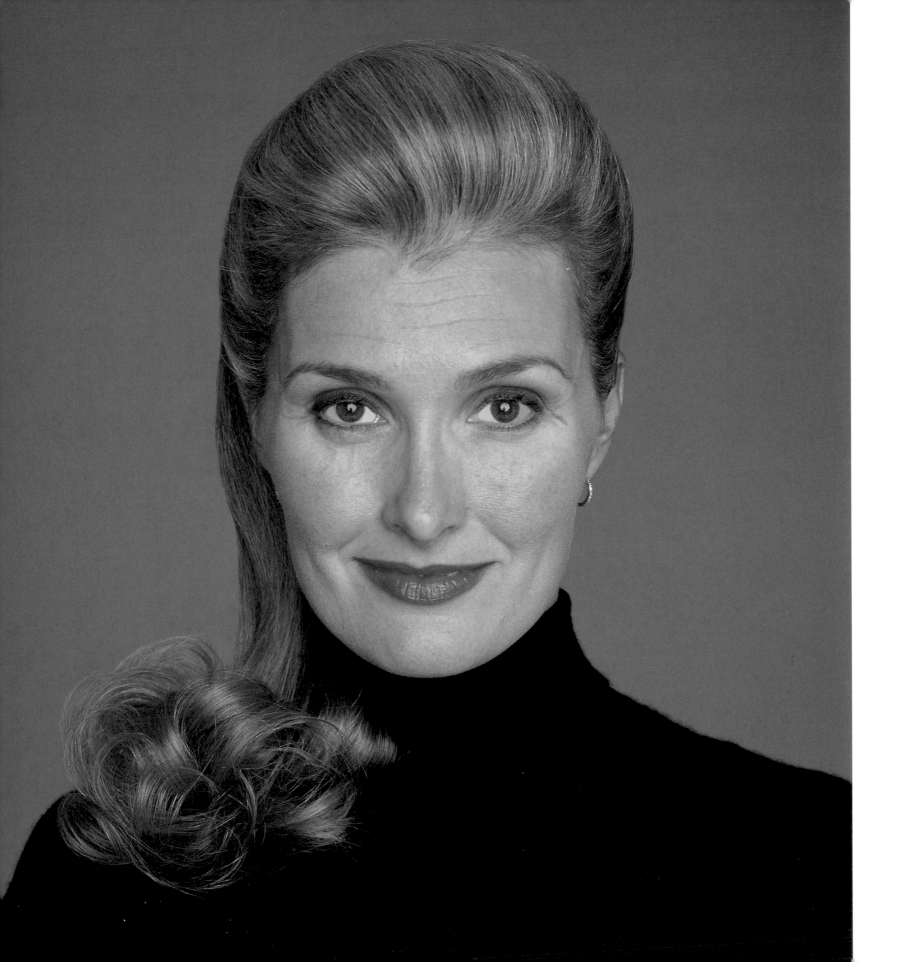

side sweep

good for

MEDIUM TO
LONG WAVY HAIR

1 Wash your hair with the shampoo of your choice, condition, towel-dry, and comb.

2 Blow-dry your hair with a round brush and rollers; set on rollers using Method 2 (see page 87). Leave the rollers in for 10 to 15 minutes and then remove gently.

3 Brush your hair out.

4 Using the top of your ear as your guide, use a comb to create an upward-slanting horizontal part on each side; gather up the hair above the part in one hand.

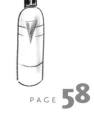

PAGE **58**

5 With that same hand, twist the hair once, then twist it again.

6 Still holding the twisted hair in the same hand, push it forward slightly to get volume into the front. Secure with bobby pins or a barrette.

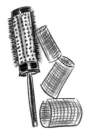

7 Brush your hair over to one side.

8 Finish with a light mist of hairspray.

PAGE **90**

PRODUCTS

Hairspray, volumizing hairspray, or shaping hairspray

TOOLS

1600-watt (or higher) blow dryer

Medium-size round brush with perforated metal cylinder

Medium-size (green) stick-on rollers

Wooden styling brush

Fine-tooth or wide-tooth comb

Bobby pins or barrette

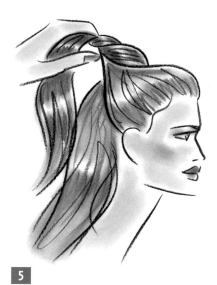

5

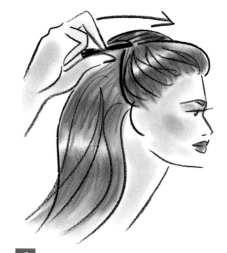

6

ALL ABOUT WAVY HAIR 133

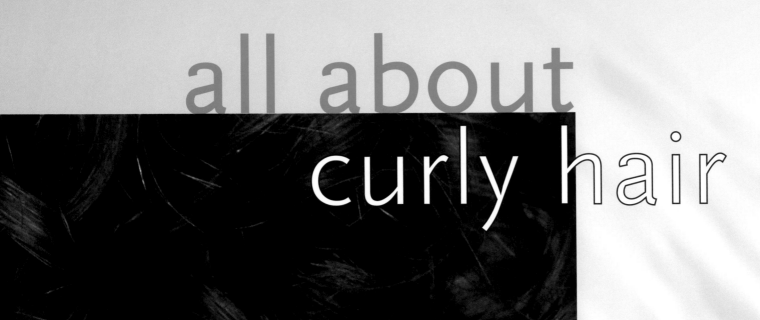

all about
curly hair

What could be prettier than rich, abundant curls? Curly hair

has lots of body and holds a style so well that you don't have

to wash it as often as other hair types.

Layered cuts work beautifully with curly hair and really bring

out its wave and curl. The shorter the layers, the tighter the

curls. If you have short hair, a basic short cut will work fine.

If you like your curls and you have a good haircut, you can let

your hair air-dry and it will look pretty good. If you want more

volume, scrunch and blow-dry it (with the diffuser sock on the

dryer) with your head flipped upside down. It's the gentle pull

of the hair away from the scalp while you're upside down that

will give the illusion of more thickness and volume.

After washing and conditioning your hair, you can comb out curly hair while it is wet. After that, though, if you're going for curl and air-drying, never comb or brush it as it dries. Once your hair is dry, keep the handling of it while styling with your fingers to a minimum. If you mess with curly hair too much as it dries and afterward, it will frizz out and your hair will end up looking like a giant powder puff.

Straightening curly hair does take some doing, and it is best accomplished by using straightening pomade, heating the hair sufficiently with the blow dryer, using the nozzle attachment for the blow dryer, creating a lot of tension with the round brush as you dry it, and using large stick-on rollers.

Common curly-hair problems are frizz and difficulty getting it to look shiny. Using shine product will help both problems and keep your hair under control on humid days.

Relaxing curly hair

A lot of people with curly hair want to relax it a bit to remove some of the tightness from the curl so that they're left with waves that are easier to blow-dry straight. This can work well, but relaxing should be done professionally or by someone with a lot of experience. It's a very risky proposition to relax your own hair unless you're quite skilled. You might break off your hair or damage it extensively.

Curly thin hair

Curls make thin hair look thicker than it actually is, which is a big plus. Volumizing products will help a lot too, but be careful not to overdo it. Using too much product will plaster your hair down, allowing others to see your scalp.

Curly thick hair

Curly thick hair can be wonderful because it is so thick and luxurious. The key is a good haircut so that your face isn't overpowered by your hair. Believe me, this is hair that can puff up and get *huge* before you know it. The downside to curly thick hair is that your scalp can get really oily if you don't use the right products. Plus, if you don't wash and rinse it properly, hair this thick will trap a lot of a product in it, leading to dull, lifeless hair and a flaky scalp. Curly thick hair also can take a long time to dry.

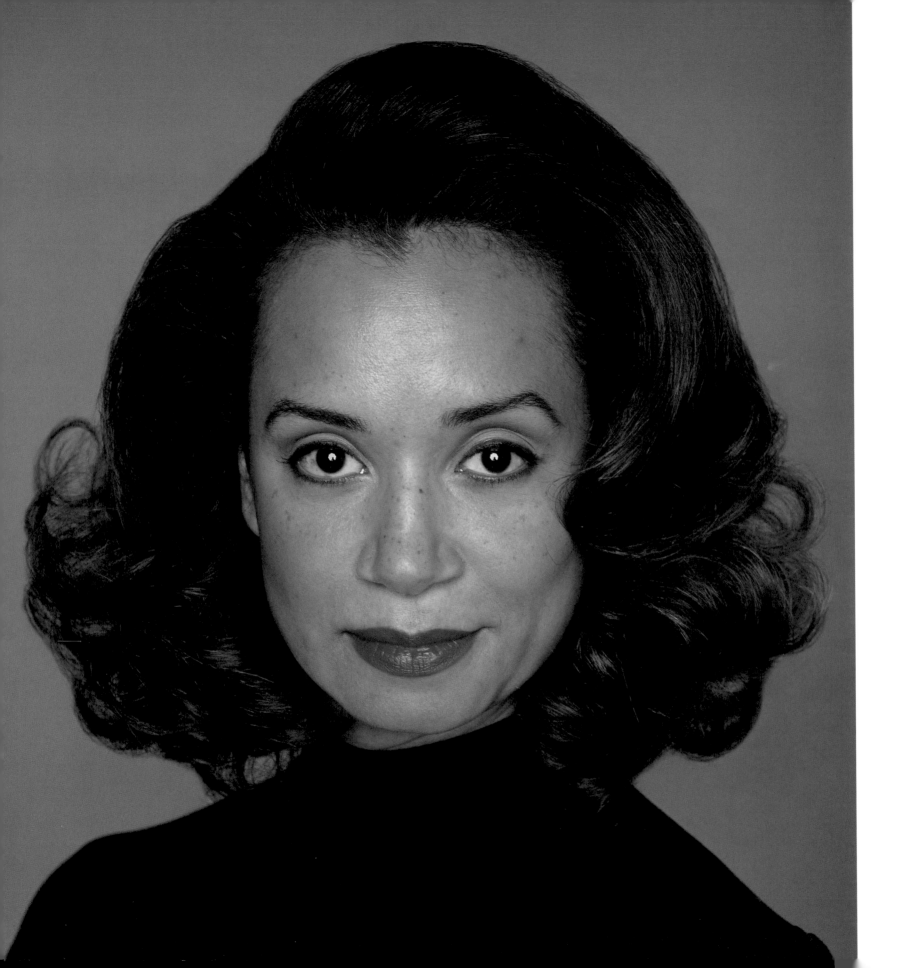

bouncy elegance

good for

SHORT TO
MEDIUM-LENGTH
CURLY HAIR

1 Wash your hair with the shampoo of your choice, condition, towel-dry, and comb.

2 Blow-dry your hair with a round brush and rollers; set on rollers using Method 1 (see page 86). Leave the rollers in for 10 to 15 minutes and then remove gently.

3 Brush your hair out.

4 Flip your head over and spray for more volume.

5 Flip your head upright. Create a part on one side with your fingers or a comb.

6 Place one hand flat on top of your head and push your hair slightly back and then forward to get lift in front. While pushing your hair forward, lightly mist the front with hairspray for a firmer hold.

7 Finish with a light mist of hairspray.

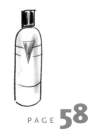

PAGE **58**

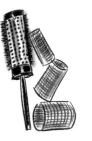

PAGE **90**

PRODUCTS

Hairspray, volumizing hairspray, or shaping hairspray

TOOLS

1600-watt (or higher) blow dryer

Medium-size round brush with perforated metal cylinder

Medium-size (green) stick-on rollers

Wooden styling brush

Fine-tooth or wide-tooth comb (optional)

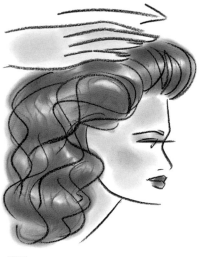

6

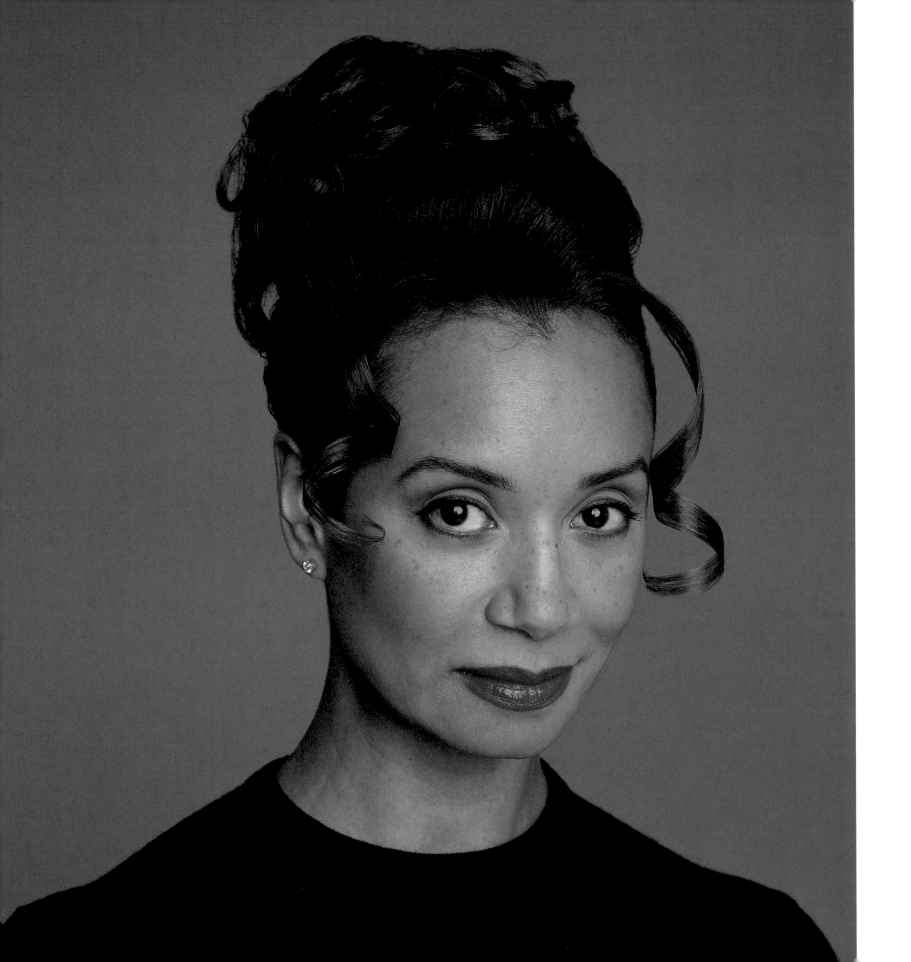

good for

SHORT TO
MEDIUM-LENGTH
CURLY HAIR

1 Wash your hair with the shampoo of your choice, condition, towel-dry, and comb.

2 Blow-dry your hair with a round brush and rollers; set on rollers using Method 2 (see page 87). Leave the rollers in for 10 to 15 minutes and then remove gently.

3 Clip aside Sections 1 and 2 and side wisps.

4 With the exception of Sections 1 and 2 and the side wisps, gather up all your hair and sweep it to the left. Insert a row of bobby pins down the center of your head, securing the hair to the side.

5 Twist the loose hair upward, forming a twist on the back of your head and leaving the ends separated on the crown.

6 Place one hand flat on top of your head and push Section 1 slightly back and then forward to get lift in front. Secure Section 1 with bobby pins. Arrange the ends from the twist and Section 2 in curls loosely on top of your head.

7 Roll each side wisp onto an extra-small (pink) roller and spray with hairspray or shaping hairspray. Leave the rollers in for 15 minutes.

8 If you have bangs, lightly back-comb them (see page 93).

9 Remove the rollers from the side wisps.

10 Finish with a light mist of hairspray.

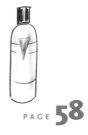

PAGE **58**

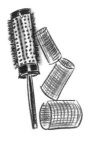

PAGE **90**

PRODUCTS

Hairspray, volumizing hairspray, or shaping hairspray

TOOLS

1600-watt (or higher) blow dryer

Medium-size round brush with perforated metal cylinder

Medium-size (green) stick-on rollers

Clips (optional)

Bobby pins

Extra-small (pink) stick-on rollers

Fine-tooth or wide-tooth comb (optional)

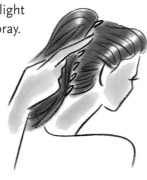

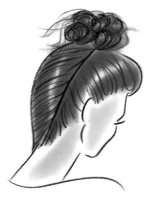

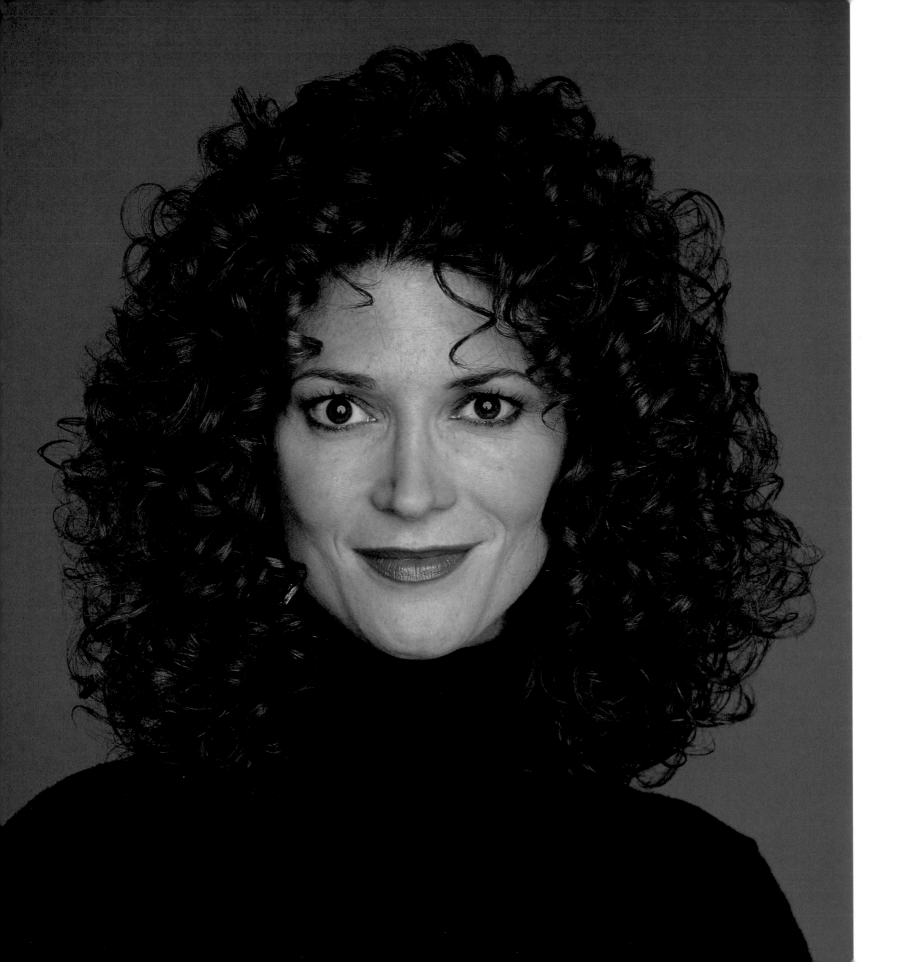

sassy curls

1 Wash your hair with the shampoo of your choice, condition, towel-dry, and comb.

2 Flip your head over. Blow-dry your hair with the diffuser sock on, being sure to scrunch the hair first. Take care not to move your hair around too much (which will cause frizzies) as you dry.

3 When your hair is completely dry, flip your head upright.

4 Gently work your fingers through your hair, lifting it away from your scalp to create volume.

5 Arrange your hair with your fingers.

6 Finish with a light mist of spray gel or hairspray.

good for

MEDIUM TO
LONG CURLY HAIR

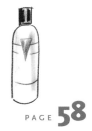

PAGE **58**

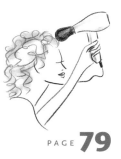

PAGE **79**

PRODUCTS

Spray gel, hairspray,
volumizing hairspray, or
shaping hairspray

TOOLS

1600-watt (or higher)
blow dryer

Diffuser sock

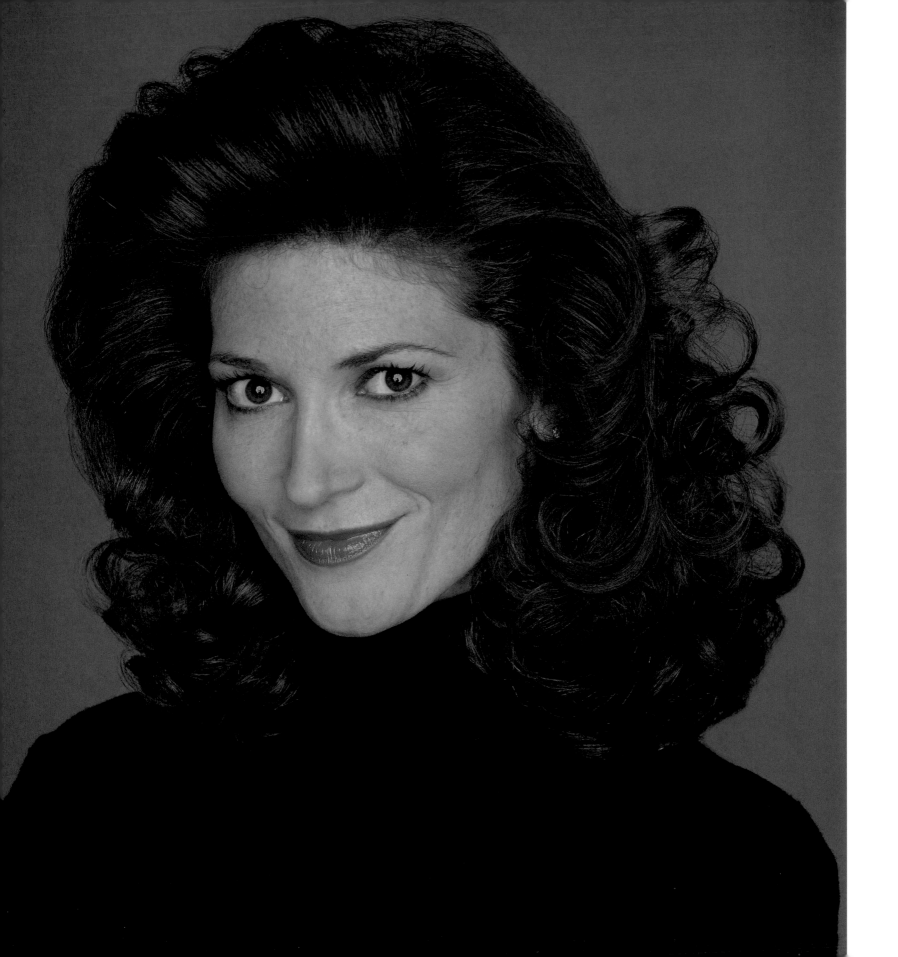

evening waves

1 Wash your hair with the shampoo of your choice, condition, towel-dry, and comb.

2 Blow-dry your hair with a round brush and rollers; set on rollers using Method 1 (see page 86). Leave the rollers in for 10 to 15 minutes and then remove gently.

3 Flip your head over and brush your hair out for volume.

4 Flip your head upright. Arrange your hair with your fingers, separating pieces to make individual curls where you want them.

5 Place one hand flat on top of your head and push your hair slightly back and then forward to get lift in front. While pushing your hair forward, lightly mist the front with hairspray for a firmer hold and lift.

6 Finish with a light mist of hairspray all over.

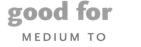

good for
MEDIUM TO LONG CURLY HAIR

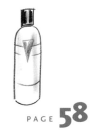

PAGE **58**

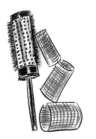

PAGE **90**

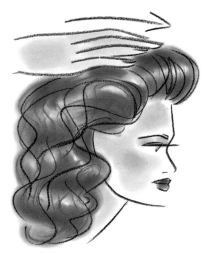

5

PRODUCTS

Hairspray, volumizing hairspray, or shaping hairspray

TOOLS

1600-watt (or higher) blow dryer

Medium-size round brush with perforated metal cylinder

Medium-size (green) stick-on rollers

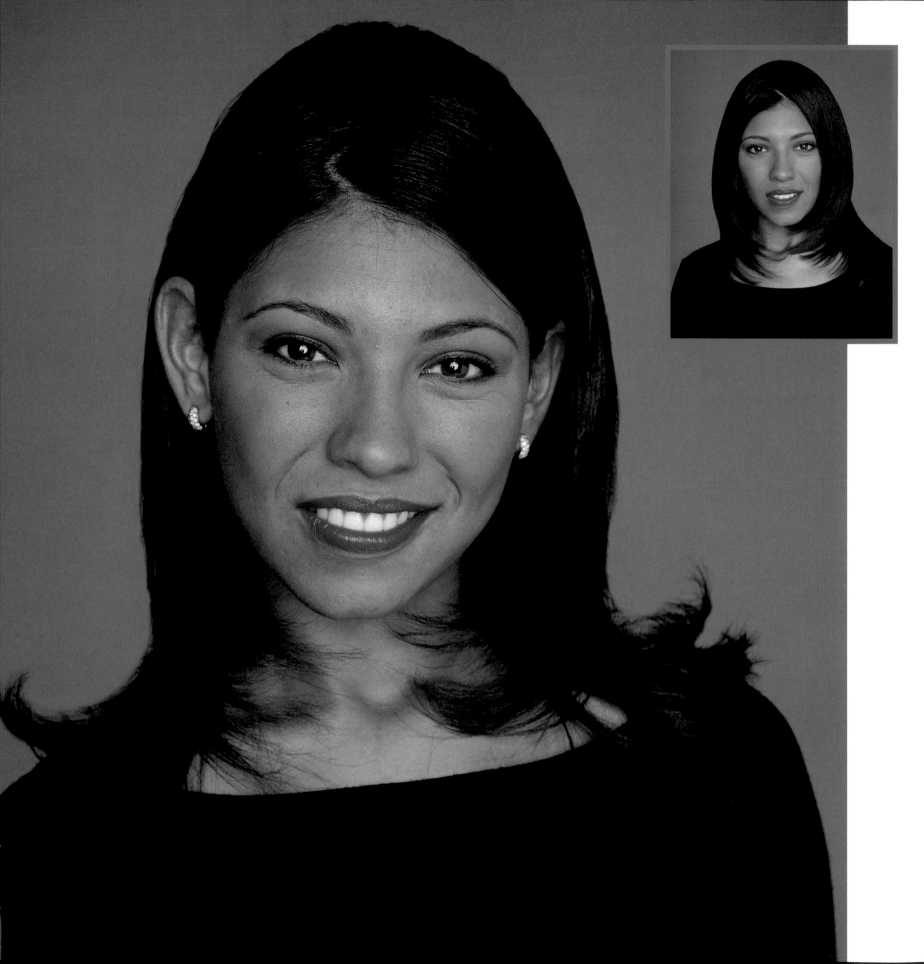

zigzag flip

good for
MEDIUM TO
LONG CURLY HAIR

1 Wash your hair with the shampoo of your choice, condition, towel-dry, and comb.

2 Blow-dry your hair with an air compressor nozzle; set on rollers using Method 1 (see page 86). Leave the rollers in for 10 to 15 minutes and then remove gently.

3 Brush your hair out.

4 Rub a drop of shine or straightening pomade into your hair to eliminate frizzies.

5 Use the end of the rat-tail comb to create a zigzag part.

6 Lightly back-comb Section 2 at the crown for added height (see page 93).

7 Flip your hair up (far left) or under (inset) at the ends (not overdirecting).

8 Finish with a light mist of hairspray.

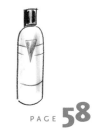

PAGE **58**

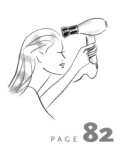

PAGE **82**

PRODUCTS

Shine or
straightening pomade

Volumizing or shaping
hairspray

TOOLS

1600-watt (or higher)
blow dryer with an air-
compressor nozzle

Medium-size round brush
with perforated metal cylinder

Medium-size (green) or
large (blue) stick-on rollers

Wooden styling brush

Rat-tail comb

all about

kinky hair

Kinky hair has a lot of body to it, but it can be frustrating for those who have it because the wiry strands grow every which way and seem to have a mind of their own. Unless it's cut very, very short, you don't want to let kinky hair air-dry.

With kinky hair, the shorter the cut, the easier it is to style. This doesn't mean you can't have long hair, but it does mean that it may take some practice to style your kinky hair the way you like.

Smoothing kinky hair

The two ways to smooth kinky hair are by blow-drying it (using heat, tension, and speed) or by wet-setting it. Once your hair is completely dry, you can also touch it up with the flattening iron if you wish.

A lot of people just blow-dry their kinky hair and keep blowing it until they singe and damage it. What you should do instead is use straightening pomade with the round brush as you blow-dry. Also, keep a spray bottle handy to dampen a section if it starts to dry and frizz up before you get a chance to dry and style it. (But be careful not to wet the sections you've already completed.)

A great trick I've found with the wet set is to blow the hair out smooth with the round brush just around the hairline first. This tames the most difficult area immediately. Then do your wet set with the largest rollers that your hair will wrap around. Once the hair is dry, finish by smoothing it out with a flattening iron or the blow dryer.

Relaxing kinky hair

For kinky, stubborn hair, relaxing is a plus. But please don't overdo it. In fact, you need to relax the hair only enough to make it a little more manageable, not poker straight. Relaxing should always be done professionally or by someone with a lot of experience. Otherwise, you risk extensive damage to your hair.

Kinky thin hair

You can see your scalp through kinky thin hair. Mousse will help, and blowing dry with the round brush is the best technique for styling it.

Kinky thick hair

Kinky thick hair can turn into a big ball. Gentle relaxing treatments are definitely a good idea. Blow-drying with a round brush or wet sets are the best techniques for styling kinky hair.

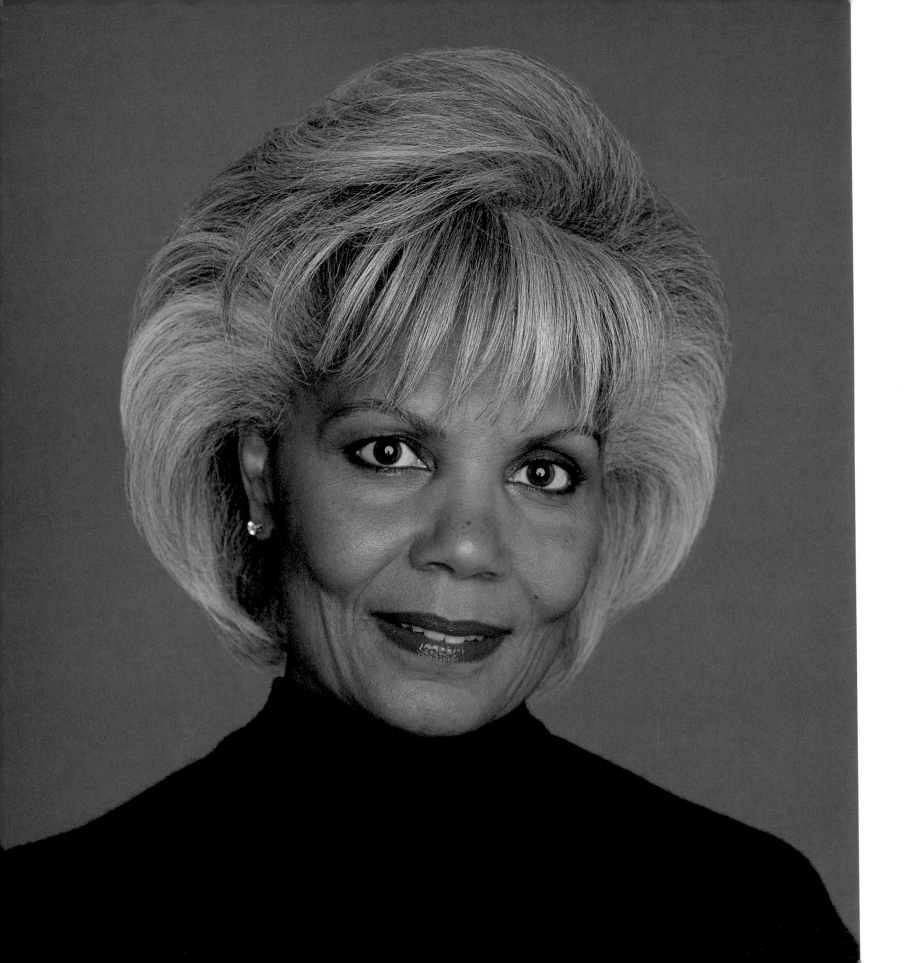

casual glamour

1 Wash your hair with the shampoo of your choice, condition, towel-dry, and comb.

2 Blow-dry your hair with a round brush and rollers; set on rollers using Method 2 (see page 87). Leave the rollers in for 10 to 15 minutes and then remove gently.

3 Brush your hair out.

4 To lift your hair away from the sides of your face, spritz spray gel or hair-spray at the roots along the temple. Brush the sprayed hair back against your head and hold it taut with the round brush. Set the blow dryer (with a diffuser sock, if you like) on a high-heat setting and point it so it blows toward the brush; heat the hair at the temple for a minute, until the spray sets.

5 Repeat Step 4 on the other side.

6 Pull your bangs forward and style with your fingers.

7 Finish with a light mist of hairspray over your whole head.

good for

SHORT TO MEDIUM-LENGTH KINKY HAIR

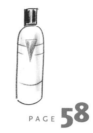

PAGE **58**

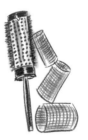

PAGE **90**

PRODUCTS

Spray gel (optional)

Hairspray or shaping hairspray

TOOLS

1600-watt (or higher) blow dryer

Medium-size round brush with perforated metal cylinder

Medium (green) stick-on rollers

Wooden styling brush

Diffuser sock (optional)

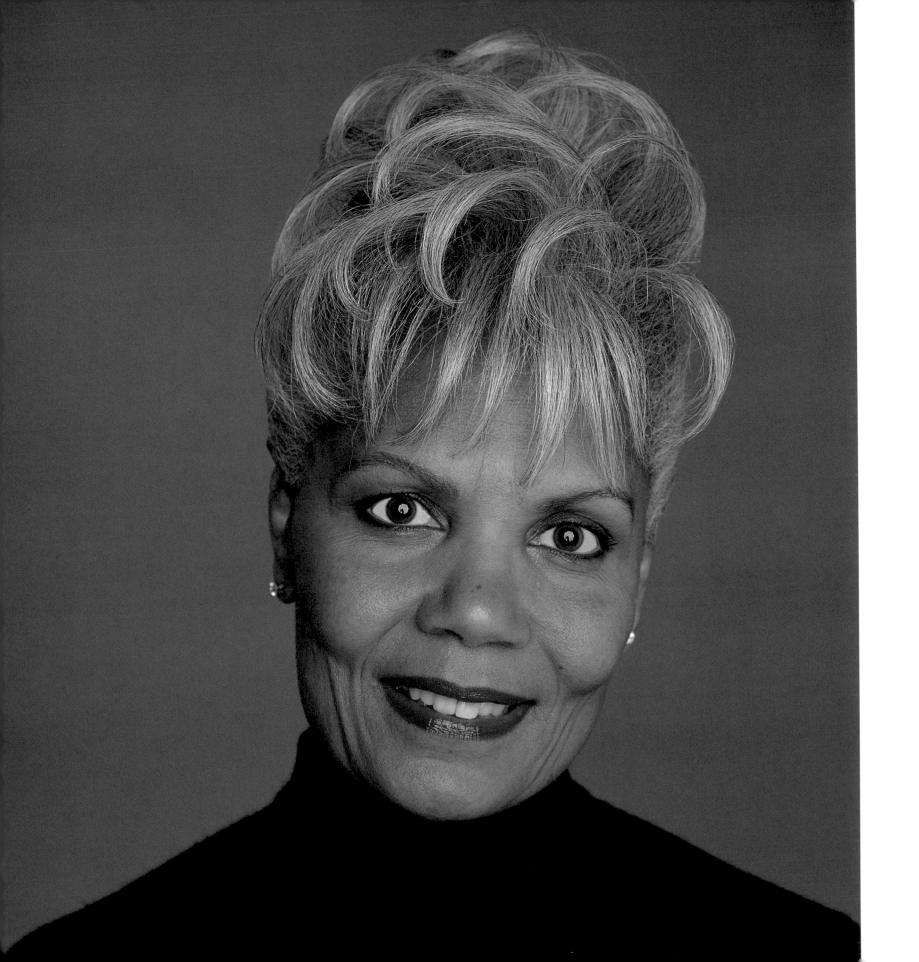

1 Wash your hair with the shampoo of your choice, condition, towel-dry, and comb.

2 Blow-dry your hair with a round brush and rollers; set on rollers using Method 2 (see page 87). Leave the rollers in for 10 to 15 minutes and then remove gently.

3 Separate Section 1 (bangs area) and Section 2 (crown) with the comb and clip them aside.

4 With the exception of Sections 1 and 2, twist the rest of your hair upward, into a French twist on the back of your head. Secure the twist with bobby pins.

5 Unclip Sections 1 and 2. At the back of Section 2, separate a small section of hair with your fingers and form it into a curl. Spray the curl with spray gel or hairspray. Place it where you want it.

6 Repeat this curl and spray process, working across the back and then toward the front and arranging the hair like petals as you go.

7 Finish with a light mist of hairspray.

good for

SHORT TO
MEDIUM-LENGTH
KINKY HAIR

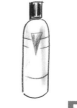

PAGE **58**

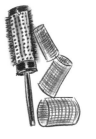

PAGE **90**

PRODUCTS

Spray gel (optional)

Hairspray or shaping hairspray

TOOLS

1600-watt (or higher) blow dryer

Medium-size round brush with perforated metal cylinder

Small (red) stick-on rollers

Fine-tooth or wide-tooth comb

Clips

Bobby pins

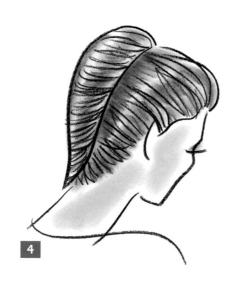

4

ALL ABOUT KINKY HAIR   155

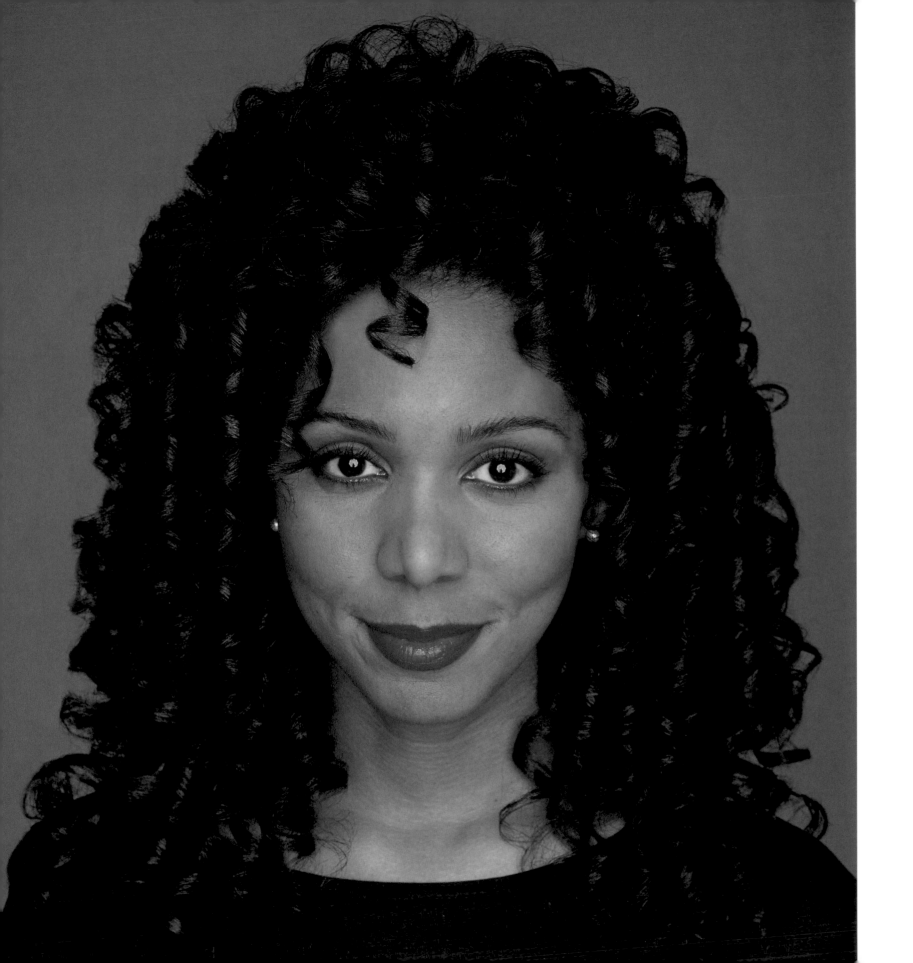

moonstruck

good for

MEDIUM TO
LONG KINKY HAIR

1 Wash your hair with the shampoo of your choice, condition, towel-dry, and comb.

2 Rub a quarter-size dollop of sculpting gel between your palms and work the gel into your hair, or thoroughly spritz your hair with spray gel.

3 Section your hair and clip in place.

4 While your hair is still damp, twist a small section around your finger, press into a pin curl, and secure with a bobby pin. Repeat until all your hair is in pin curls. If your hair dries before you pin-curl it, slightly wet it again with water from a spray bottle.

5 Dry your hair using a blow dryer with diffuser sock or a hooded dryer.

6 After your hair is completely dry, unpin and release the curls. Do not brush.

7 Separate the coil of each curl by pulling it apart with your fingers to create smaller and more abundant curls.

8 Arrange your hair with your fingers.

9 Finish with a light mist of hairspray.

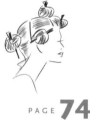

PAGE **58**

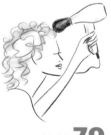

PAGE **74**

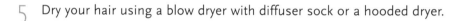

PAGE **79**

PRODUCTS

Sculpting gel or spray gel

Hairspray or shaping hairspray

TOOLS

Clips

Bobby pins

Spray bottle of water (optional)

1600-watt (or higher) blow dryer with diffuser sock or hooded dryer

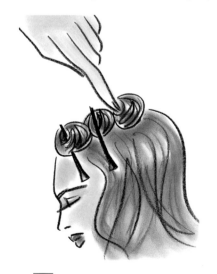

4

cascading curls

1 Wash your hair with the shampoo of your choice, condition, towel-dry, and comb.

2 Set your wet hair on rollers using Method 1 (see page 86) and dry under a hooded dryer on high setting for 30 to 45 minutes, depending on the thickness of your hair. If you don't have access to a hooded dryer, use a blow dryer with a diffuser sock. When your hair is completely dry, allow it to cool for 10 to 15 minutes and then gently remove the rollers.

3 Brush your hair out.

4 Lightly spritz spray gel or hairspray at the hairline or anywhere else there are frizzies, ridges, or roller marks. Using a round brush, push those areas down against your hairline. Roll frizzy or problem areas onto the round brush and warm with a blast of heat from the blow dryer on a high-heat setting.

5 Finish with a light mist of hairspray.

good for

MEDIUM TO
LONG KINKY HAIR

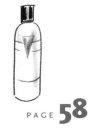

PAGE **58**

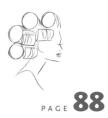

PAGE **88**

PRODUCTS

Spray gel (optional)

Hairspray or shaping hairspray

TOOLS

Large (blue) stick-on rollers

Hooded dryer (or a blow dryer with a diffuser sock)

Wooden styling brush

Medium-size round brush with perforated metal cylinder

Afterword

I feel that I have been given many gifts in my life—a wonderful and loving family, a deep belief in God, and the opportunity to do something professionally that makes people happy and feel good about themselves.

Writing this book has been a true pleasure for me because it's a real opportunity to give back, not only to my wonderful clients and customers but literally everyone, the knowledge, advice, and experience, that I have acquired over a lifetime.

And I know this information can work for you and help you enhance the beauty that is already uniquely yours!

God bless,

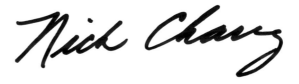